Communicating through Movement

Sherborne Developmental Movement –
towards a broadening perspective

Cyndi Hill

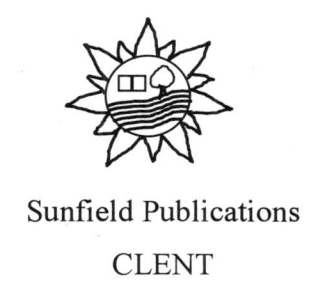

Sunfield Publications
CLENT

The right of the author to be identified as author of this work has been asserted by them in accordance with the Copyright, Designs and Patents Act 1988.

Copyright © Cyndi Hill 2006

First published in Great Britain
by Sunfield Publications 2006.

Published by
Sunfield Publications
Sunfield, Woodman Lane, Clent, Stourbridge DY9 9PB.

ISBN: 0-9550568-0-2

All rights reserved. No part of this publication may be reproduced in any material form (including photocopying or storing it in any medium by electronic means and whether or not transiently or incidentally to some other use of this publication) without the written permission of the copyright owner except in accordance with the provisions of the Copyright, Designs and Patents Act 1988. Applications for the copyright owner's written permission to reproduce any part of this publication should be addressed to the publisher.

Warning: The doing of an unauthorised act in relation to a copyright work may result in both a civil claim for damages and criminal prosecution.

Printed and bound in Great Britain by
PCL WOLLASTON PRINT LIMITED
Richmond House, Richmond Road, Smethwick, West Midlands B66 4ED.

For

Michael George

'We celebrate your life.'

Author's note

I have wanted to write such a book as this for several years, but to have started it any earlier, I now know, would have been a mistake. I have long felt the need for some form of theoretical support for Veronica Sherborne's work, but there have been so many developments in the field of education, therapy and care in recent years, and I have learnt so much between the time when I first thought about 'writing a book' and now, that I am glad I did not start writing sooner.

I have had time to consider in more depth what it is I want to say about Sherborne Developmental Movement (SDM), and I have learnt a tremendous amount through my continuing work both with children and adults, and through shared conversations with other Sherborne colleagues since the setting up of The Sherborne Association UK.

I envisage this book as being of interest to teachers, classroom support workers, psychologists, therapists, social workers and people who work in the community – all those whose work may include focusing on 'supporting people with disabilities of any kind'.

I see its readership as falling into two main categories: firstly, those who already have an awareness of Sherborne's work, are familiar with the basic principles of SDM and wish to extend their perception of the work; and, secondly, those who are viewing its contents from the broader perspective as a means of 'communication' and who might subsequently wish to pursue further knowledge through attending courses and reading Sherborne's book, *Developmental Movement for Children* (Sherborne, 2001).

Contents

	Page no.
Acknowledgements	vi
Contributing Authors	viii
Foreword	x
Introduction	xii

Part One: The Evolving Theory

Chapter 1	Veronica Sherborne: Biographical Notes and the Laban Influence	2
Chapter 2	The Evolving Theory: Philosophical and Theoretical Aspects which Underpin Sherborne Developmental Movement	7
Chapter 3	Psychological, Educational and Sociological Implications	19

Part Two: From Theory into Practice

Chapter 4	Practical Aspects of a Sherborne Developmental Movement Session	35
Chapter 5	Sherborne Developmental Movement in the Community and in Therapy	51
Chapter 6	Sherborne Developmental Movement in Education	82

Part Three: Questions and Projects

Chapter 7	Some Frequently Asked Questions, with Answers and Suggestions	101
Chapter 8	The Sherborne Developmental Movement/Science Project	108
Chapter 9	Research Projects: Recent and On-going	112
Chapter 10	A Concluding Summary	123

Appendices	126
Index	156

Acknowledgements

My thanks are due to the many, many people who have taken an interest, given me support, and contributed towards this project.

Firstly, I would like to thank Sarah Sherborne for the good wishes and encouragement which she gave me when I first approached her about the writing of this book.

My thanks to Stephen Morris, the head teacher, and the staff, pupils and students of Warmley Park School (formerly Grimsbury Park School), who have been part of my 'Sherborne experience' for so many years, and who participated in the action research project which I describe in Chapter 9. Along with them, I would also like to thank Julie Kembry, a parent/governor of the school, who acted as one of my 'observers' for that project.

My husband, George Hill, who with me has shared an interest in Sherborne's work over the years, has had many roles in the process of producing this book. Along with Julie Kembry, he was also an 'observer' for the action research project. I wrote the bulk of Chapter 4 based on his notes and observations concerning the practical application of Sherborne Developmental Movement (SDM), and he also supplied me with information about his work with students at Bristol University and about using SDM as a team-building activity. Perhaps he has shown his greatest fortitude in helping me through the numerous computing processes required to produce the original script, and, for his help in that respect, I am particularly grateful.

I am especially indebted to the people who contributed towards Chapter 5. My thanks go to Dr. Janice Filer, for her account of her early intervention programme, Developmental Movement Play, and to Penny Rance for writing about her work with Dance in the Community for young people with varying difficulties. For a physiotherapist's view of SDM in the UK, my thanks go to Chris Handley, a senior chartered physiotherapist, who is attached to a special school in Staffordshire. I feel I must say a special word of thanks to my Belgian colleagues, Ilse Bontinck, Nathalie Vanassche, Danny Dossche, Ingeborg Vandamme, Marlene Van Rentergem and Kurt Fierens, who not only related how they incorporate SDM into their therapeutic settings, but also did so using a 'second language'. I really do appreciate the additional effort which this must have entailed.

To my friends and colleagues in The Sherborne Association, I would like to say 'thank you' for their encouragement and support for this project. My thanks go to Margaret Vinson, who shared with me her thoughts on the work of Feuerstein and his Instrumental Enrichment Programme, and to Janet Sparkes, Dr Elizabeth Marsden and Bill Richards, for supplying me with information about their use of SDM with students in higher education. In addition, Dr Marsden has also provided me with an overview of a research project in which she was involved with teachers and pupils in a mainstream setting in Kent.

An outline of on-going research, which is being undertaken collaboratively between Sunfield School in the West Midlands and The Sherborne Association UK has been kindly provided by Jotham Konaka, who is leading the project. I must add to that a special word of thanks to Bill Richards, who proofread my original script with such obvious diligence and care, and offered me so much sound, helpful and constructive advice.

I would also like to thank my friend and colleague, Bjarne Dahl, for reading my script and making valuable suggestions, which I have since incorporated into the title and content of this book. Bjarne was among the first group of Norwegians to meet Veronica Sherborne, and subsequently to work with her in Norway.

I feel it is probably true to say that this book would not have come to into being without the support and encouragement which I have received from Professor Barry Carpenter, the chief executive and director of research at Sunfield School. I would like to thank him, not only for writing the Foreword, but also for his help with the publication of the book itself, and for his personal commitment and effort to maintain the continuation and development of Sherborne's work. For her support and energy in actually getting this publication to print, my thanks go to Rose Welling. To Jo Egerton, who copy-edited my typescript, for her unfailing encouragement and meticulous advice throughout the whole process, I am sincerely grateful.

My final thanks must go to my own family – to my husband, George, whom I have already mentioned, to our daughters, Helen, Carolyn (who has helped me in particular with many of the computing techniques), Debra and Karen, all of whom have always supported me and taken an interest in my work, and, lastly, to our son, Michael George who, throughout his shortened life, provided inspiration for us all. To Michael George I dedicate this book.

Contributing Authors

Chapter 5
Dr Janice Filer, a teacher trained in physical education and dance, describes how she incorporates Sherborne Developmental Movement (SDM) into her innovative early intervention programme, Developmental Movement Play, with parents and young children who may be experiencing problems with communication, relationships, and emotional, behavioural and mental health difficulties.

Penny Rance is a community dance worker who specialises in leading workshops for people with physical and/or learning disabilities. She is an 'arts worker', rather than a therapist, by background, training and choice. She works with children and adults in a wide variety of settings, mostly leading regular dance sessions, interspersed with short-term projects and one-off sessions. A recent, exciting development for her has been her involvement in training and mentoring other interested dance workers in working with people with disabilities.

Danny Dossche and *Ingeborg Vandamme* (physiotherapists), *Ilse Bontinck* and *Nathalie Vanassche* (occupational therapists) and *Marleen Van Rentergem* and *Kurt Fierens* (speech and language therapists), work in a 'readaptation centre' in Deinze, Belgium. They work with developmentally delayed children, who have varying needs, in a multidisciplinary team under the supervision of a psychologist and a paediatric doctor. They use SDM, not only as part of their individual therapy treatment, but also as a basis for their multidisciplinary team involvement, in which they adopt an holistic approach to work with children who attend their centre.

Chris Handley is a senior chartered physiotherapist who is involved in work with pupils and students who attend a special school in Staffordshire. Her contribution, by way of 'A physiotherapist's view of Sherborne Developmental Movement' sets her use of Sherborne's ideas within the context of her overall work in the field of physiotherapy in this particular setting in the UK.

Chapter 6
Janet Sparkes has recently retired from full time lecturing at the University of Winchester, but continues to contribute to aspects of teacher training. She has used Sherborne Developmental Movement with both children and adults over many years in different situations, including a variety of contexts in Romania.

Bill Richards is a Physical Education specialist who has taught in secondary, primary and special schools. Between 1984 and 2001, he lectured in Physical Education and Teacher Education at the University of Plymouth. Since 2001, he has been an educational consultant at Vranch House School and Centre in Exeter

Chapters 4 and 6
George Hill has had a varied, interesting and rewarding career. Starting in the Royal Air Force as an electronics engineer, he moved to the Prison Service as the long-term allocation officer. From there, he became the manager of a large Training Centre for adults with disabilities. He then moved on to resettling hospital residents into the community and finally became an inspector of residential homes. During the latter part of his career, he met and worked closely with Veronica Sherborne. He helped to found The Sherborne Association and took her work into Finland, Estonia and Japan, as well as working in other European Countries.

Chapters 6 and 9
Dr Elizabeth Marsden is currently course leader for Physical Education at the University of Paisley, Scotland, where she tries to inspire primary student teachers to approach Physical Education creatively. She worked alongside Veronica Sherborne for many years and is now examining her philosophy and claims through present-day research

Chapter 9
Jotham Konaka is a teacher/researcher with over 20 years teaching experience in the area of special educational needs. He is currently working at Sunfield School for children with severe and complex learning difficulties, including Autistic Spectrum Disorders (ASD). Jotham is a strong believer in promoting intervention strategies that can provide curriculum access to individuals with learning difficulties and improve their personal learning profiles. As a founder member of the Special Schools Sports Association of Kenya, he contributed immensely towards the development of a Physical Education curriculum for children with physical and neurological disabilities in the country. He is currently exploring the use of SDM to support social engagement with children with severe ASD as part of his doctorate studies.

Foreword

During the rapid formative period of special education in the late 1960s and 1970s, Veronica Sherborne was a towering influence. Her Developmental Movement enabled many teachers, confronted with children previously unseen in special schools (or even the education system), to engage meaningfully with these children. Her unique approach facilitated communication, encouraged interaction, stimulated physical activity, and developed relationships. Indeed, 'relationship play' was another term Sherborne used for her Developmental Movement.

The concept of 'relationship play' bridged, for many teachers, the worlds of Early Childhood (Infant) Education in which they had been trained and the new world of special education where children presented with severe, profound and complex needs. What curriculum would meet these needs? Were infant teaching methods appropriate? What pedagogy would be responsive to the challenges posed by these children? Sherborne proved, time and time again, that the elements of her programme enabled children to acquire relevant skills, establish meaningful relationships, and, most of all, enjoy the process.

Veronica Sherborne was a charismatic character. As a newly qualified teacher working in a special school, I encountered Veronica on an HMI-led course. I was immediately captivated by the capacity of the Developmental Movement programme to meet the needs of the children in my class. The responsive nature of Sherborne Developmental Movement (SDM) has been proved time and time again for me in its capacity to include children with wide-ranging special educational needs.

Sherborne was not much inclined to write down her thoughts, but finally, in 1990, *Developmental Movement for Children* was published. It was reprinted in 2001. Much has changed in education generally, and special education specifically, since the first edition was published. The context today is very different to the one in which Veronica Sherborne developed the programme, yet practitioners using SDM testify time and time again to its effectiveness with children. It has met the challenges of emerging groups, such as children with profound and multiple learning difficulties (PMLD), and has shown its capacity to support the development of the current burgeoning group of children – those with autistic spectrum disorders. (Research reported in this text discusses this area in more detail.)

However, the need for SDM to be recast into a present-day, educational context which includes the National Curriculum, Individual Education Plans, Care Standards, and moves towards inclusive education, is pressing. Cyndi Hill, also a former student of Veronica Sherborne, has risen to this challenge magnificently in *Communicating through Movement*.

This work is firmly rooted in the seminal text, *Developmental Movement for Children*. In this book, Veronica Sherborne articulated her theoretical, philosophical and practical approach to Developmental Movement. Most of all, her fascination with its impact on, and benefits for, children with a whole range of special educational needs is obvious for all to see. The pivotal tenet in SDM is its capacity for engagement – a fundamental, underpinning concept in all aspects of special education. To see the disturbed and disturbing child liberated from the confines of their disability and engage with another human being, interacting and communicating, is truly breath-taking. This is the power of SDM.

Cyndi Hill writes with passion and conviction of the facilitating powers of SDM, and its capacity to meet the holistic needs of the child with special educational needs, in ways that many other curriculum areas cannot replicate or achieve. From a thorough discussion of the influences, theories and philosophies embodied in SDM, she moves to a rich section on the practical aspects of SDM. These chapters (4–6), combined with the information-rich observation and recording sheets in the Appendices, will be greatly valued by practitioners in a variety of settings.

The final part of the book effectively pulls together frequently asked questions, and provides useful answers. Chapter 9 shows how research can be undertaken with SDM. This approach to evidence-based practice is crucial to answering the many questions posed by the ever-changing population of children and adults with special educational needs. These examples show the dynamic nature of SDM. It is not a static programme locked in a time-warp. It is a constantly evolving, child-centred approach, which effectively and meaningfully meets children at their point of need.

Cyndi Hill has ensured that SDM is brought into the 21st Century, and, through her deep commitment, has demonstrated its relevance for children today, as Veronica Sherborne did two decades ago. Through detailing the programme in the current curriculum context, she ensures that children, and the staff working with them, have access to this vibrant and vital approach to teaching and learning. Her passion pervades her writing, giving it life and energy.

This book will do much to bring SDM to the attention of practitioners in a range of settings. I commend it to you.

Barry Carpenter, OBE
Sunfield, Clent, Worcestershire
September 2005

Introduction

I was initially introduced to 'Sherborne Movement' in 1971, through my work as a teacher, when I moved from a mainstream primary setting into the field of special education. I attended four one-day workshops led by Veronica Sherborne, and was inspired by the apparent simplicity and basic, down-to-earth characteristics of her work and the way she presented her ideas. On returning to school, I immediately began to try some of those ideas with my class group, and have continued to be involved with Sherborne's work, in varying roles, ever since. Two years later, Veronica also taught my husband, who at that time was working with adults with special needs. He recognised the benefits her work could offer his people, and began to use her ideas at his adult training centre.

As we lived on the outskirts of Bristol, not too far from Veronica, we were to see her on many occasions in the future. I would take groups of our children to work with her students at the then Bristol Polytechnic; she would bring visitors, often from abroad, to my school to see her ideas in action. We would visit her quite frequently to talk about her work and our involvement in it, and, towards the end of her life when she had been persuaded finally to spend time on writing a book, she had already begun asking us to lead courses for her, at first in the UK and then abroad.

In the course of our travels, around the world and in the UK where we have been invited to lead courses and workshops on Sherborne Developmental Movement (SDM), we have heard the words, 'It works!' so many times. In the vast majority of cases, given the right environment and circumstances, it does – but *why* does it work?

It is not enough simply to make subjective statements concerning the values and benefit of using SDM. As practitioners, we need not only to have a subjective knowledge of the practical aspects of the work, but we also need to be able to rationalise the work. Sarah Sherborne, writing in the preface to the second edition of her mother's book (Sherborne, 2001), points out that her mother was a 'do-er', a very practical person, and Sherborne herself would repeatedly point out that:

> *People have to 'do' my movement to fully understand its true value, and to 'feel' the effect of the movements for themselves.**

In an unpublished paper, now housed with the Sherborne archive material, which can be accessed through The Sherborne Association UK, she writes:

> *... it is important that the movements are seen as bodily experiences and not as mechanical exercises. We need to become as deeply involved as possible in what we are doing, otherwise the activities will be superficial and have little meaning or value.* (Sherborne, 1979)

She had an unflinching belief in her work, often striving against the influential thinking of the time. However, during the years which have elapsed between the publication of her book in 1990 and the present time, her work has not only become accepted in many fields beyond that of education, in which she mostly developed her ideas, but there have also evolved significant issues and requirements which now need to be addressed.

Among those issues and requirements, there is now a need for objective analysis and theoretical enquiry in order to give the work credibility for the future. Recognising this requirement, Janet Sparkes, writing on behalf of The Sherborne Association UK, in the Foreword to the second edition of Veronica's book, makes reference to the 'evolving theory' (Sherborne, 2001, p. xi). That the essence of the work must remain subjective in its implementation is absolutely imperative, but, at the same time, the work must stand up to objective scrutiny. This dual approach to Sherborne's work has been fundamental to my thinking and decisions concerning the format and content of this book.

For this reason, I have come to the conclusion that I also need to reflect both the inherent subjectivity of individual approaches to SDM together with objective investigation within this book. Some of the frames of reference I use are based on my personal contact and conversations with Veronica, others on my personal experience of using SDM in varying contexts – both as a practising teacher and as a course leader. Other frames of reference are literature-based, where my purpose is to find academic support to substantiate various aspects of Sherborne's work.

Although some readers will want to read this book from cover to cover, I anticipate that many will want to 'dip into' different sections. For this reason, I have repeated some material to provide an immediate context for more than one section.

In Part 1, where the emphasis is on the theory which underpins Sherborne's work, I use an objective, academically based style, whereas in Part 2, which describes the practical aspects and application of SDM, and the use of Sherborne's ideas in varying contexts, the style becomes much more subjective. These varying writing styles, far from detracting from the text as a whole, I feel, reflect the breadth and richness of Sherborne's work across a very wide spectrum. This is enhanced by the fact that part of Chapter 5 is written by Belgian colleagues, who, it must be remembered, are writing in a 'second language'. In Part 3, which is made up of my personal responses to questions, and reports on projects that I have undertaken, I endeavour to use a 'descriptive' style of writing. Each of these different writing styles is totally appropriate to SDM within the varying contexts of its application, whilst at the same time reflecting the 'broadening perspective' referred to in the subtitle of this book.

Part 1
The opening chapter provides a brief biographical background to the life and work of Veronica Sherborne, a testimony to her constant acknowledgement of

the influence of Rudolf Laban on her work, and lastly describes the setting up of The Sherborne Association in her memory. It is based on information gained from conversations with Veronica (and kindly verified by her daughter, Sarah Sherborne), and my personal involvement with The Sherborne Association UK.

Chapter 2 outlines what I see as theories and ideas which contribute to the 'evolving theory' which underpins the practice of SDM. This is based on my work with Sherborne, the reading of her papers, watching her films and videos, and the study of her book, *Developmental Movement for Children* (Sherborne, 2001). In latter years, I have also had the privilege of taking part in many enriching discussions with colleagues in Sherborne Associations in the UK and abroad.

It is my belief that, although the implementation of Sherborne's work is, in essence, 'simple', there are, embodied within the work, profoundly significant, psychological influences which can greatly affect the development of those taking part in SDM sessions in a very positive and beneficial way. As Sherborne says in the introduction to her book:

> *The activities described in this book are referred to as 'experiences' rather than 'exercises', because they combine both physical and psychological learning experiences.* (Sherborne, 2001, p. xiv)*

Chapter 3, therefore, looks objectively at perspectives which support Sherborne's work – using published psychological, educational, sociological and developmental material – and relates aspects of SDM to the 'teaching and learning' process and theories of personality development.

Part 2

Returning to the more practical aspects of the work, Chapter 4 discusses the preparation and planning of movement sessions, and ways in which details of this planning may vary according to the diverse needs of the participants.

Recognising that Sherborne's ideas are now being used in a much wider field than that of education, Chapter 5 is included as an 'invitation chapter' written by practitioners who are using Sherborne's work in varying therapeutic environments, including physiotherapy, speech and language therapy, occupational therapy, and community dance with families in a socially challenged area.

Although the professional spectrum of interest in Sherborne's work is broadening considerably, the main focus of interest still remains, at this time, in the fields of pre-school and special education. With this in mind, using the National Curriculum and related documents as the main reference, Chapter 6 highlights some of the many ways in which SDM can support the teaching of core subjects, and cross-references SDM activities to UK National Curriculum requirements. I have also in this chapter addressed the concept of 'inclusion', as

I feel that SDM can make a very valuable contribution in this area, not only within the curriculum, but also from its philosophical perspective.

Sherborne originally used her movement ideas with students who were undergoing training to become teachers of children with learning difficulties. With this in mind, Sherborne Association colleagues who have used SDM with students attending courses in higher education have written the concluding part of this chapter.

Part 3
When presenting courses on SDM, I find that there are questions which are frequently asked. Some of these questions will already have been addressed elsewhere in the book, but, in Chapter 7, I have summarised them and offered some suggestions and answers.

Chapter 8 is an account of an SDM/Science project, which I ran at a school for pupils and students with severe learning difficulties, in which we explored some of the properties of light and sound through movement, science activities and dance.

The final chapter is an account of a classroom-based action research project, which I undertook recently, to investigate the possible effect of SDM sessions on subsequent classroom behaviour. Using schedules designed to record specific designated behaviours in terms of 'concentration and attention' and 'social interaction', observations were made in the classroom, and then repeated in the same classroom settings, using exactly the same procedures, but immediately following a movement session. I have also included reports of recent research projects, one of which explores the use of SDM in a mainstream setting, whilst the other investigates the use of SDM as a way of increasing social engagement with pupils who have autistic spectrum disorder.

In compiling this book, I have had three main objectives in mind. Firstly, in Part 1, to explore 'the evolving theory', and then, from the present-day consensus of psychological, educational and sociological thinking, to find theories which substantiate and support Sherborne's ideas and way of working. My second objective, reflected in Part 2 and bearing in mind the subtitle of the book, 'towards a broadening perspective', is to explore some of the uses of Sherborne's work in various community and therapeutic settings, and to reiterate its continuing value within the present-day educational system. Within this framework, there are issues addressed that were not as predominant when Sherborne was writing in 1990 as they are at the present time, and which, therefore, I feel now need to be considered. In Part 3, I share some of my personal experiences with SDM, and endeavour to answer some of the questions that are regularly asked concerning the implementation of Sherborne's work.

The work of Veronica Sherborne through SDM, which depends intrinsically on the nature and quality of the interaction between the participants, does not readily lend itself to verbal or written description. Indeed, it was not until 1990, shortly before her death, that her own book, *Developmental Movement for Children,* was first published. Having said that, however, literature support there must be for those who recognise the potential of her work and wish to see it continued into the future. Referring again to the Foreword of the second edition of Sherborne's book, I can most certainly relate to the statement that:

> *Those who worked and studied with Veronica Sherborne can not fail to have been impressed by the dynamic quality of the learning experience she created.* (Sparkes, in Sherborne, 2001, p. xi)*

This was most certainly the case for me, and I hope that this book will in some way help to perpetuate the use of Veronica Sherborne's unique and invaluable ideas, which are encapsulated in what we now refer to as Sherborne Developmental Movement.

References
Sherborne, V. (1979) Sherborne Movement (Unpublished paper).
Sherborne, V. (2001) *Developmental Movement for Children: Mainstream, special needs and pre-school* (2nd edn). London: Worth Publishing.

*Reprinted by kind permission of Worth Publishing from *Developmental Movement for Children* by Veronica Sherborne.
2nd Edition. Worth Publishing Limited 2001.

PART 1

The Evolving Theory

CHAPTER 1
Veronica Sherborne:
Biographical Notes and the Laban Influence

In her classroom we were all equal. Her work was based on the clear recognition of the power and intelligence of the human spirit, beyond disability. She enabled us all to be physically strong, playful and capable of helping each other. (Hodgson, 1991)

These words, for me, encapsulate beautifully, succinctly and accurately the work of Veronica Sherborne. Developed over a period of 30 years – during which she placed great importance on observing her own three children, and working with children and adults with varying needs in a variety of situations, with their parents, teachers, care workers and therapists – her unique way of working focuses on a framework of shared movement experiences.

She trained initially at Bedford College of Physical Education as a teacher of Physical Education and Dance. Her first post was at Cheltenham Ladies College in Gloucestershire, where she stayed for three years. However, whilst still training at Bedford, she had her first encounter with Rudolf Laban – an experience that was to have a profound effect on the rest of her professional life.

Such was the influence of this two-day encounter with Laban that, in 1946, she relinquished her post at Cheltenham Ladies College to study for two years at Lisa Ullman's Art of Movement Studio in Manchester, where Laban was a lecturer. It would appear that she was somewhat outstanding as a student as, after completing the course, she was invited to stay on and work with Laban, who acknowledged her contribution to his work in the Introduction to his book, *Modern Educational Dance* (1948).

Rudolf Laban, born in Bratislava in 1879, had come to England in 1938 as a refugee from Germany, where his work had been branded as '"against the state", being regarded as not sufficiently nationalistic' (Thornton, 1971). Laban's movement analysis and his philosophy surrounding 'dance' is a vast, well-researched subject, which has had a significant influence on many forms of movement in this country; his term, 'free-dance', encapsulates its underlying principals.

Laban was interested in the dancer's free expression of the inner self and feelings. He is quoted as saying:

If you saw several of my students dance you would never guess that they were trained by the same man. (Laban, cited in Thornton, 1971, p. 21)

In *Modern Educational Dance*, Laban suggests that:

> ...*a refreshing swim in the sea is a wonderful, health-giving thing... It is a very similar case with the occasional swim in the flow of movement... [As] water is a widespread means of sustaining life, so too is the flow of movement.* (Laban, 1948, p. 97)

In very simple terms, in order to be able to take this 'occasional swim in the flow of movement', we need to have confidence in our own bodies and how we move, an awareness of space in all its dimensions, an awareness of 'movement qualities', and the confidence to make positive relationships. What part of the body is moving, where in space it is moving, and how it is moving are some of the key considerations in Laban's movement analysis. In terms of 'space', he was interested in high space, low space, space to each side, moving forwards into space in front, and backwards into space behind. He taught that 'pathways through space', in terms of direct (straight) and flexible (curving) lines, concentrate the thinking on 'travelling through space'.

Awareness of Laban's movement qualities, in addition to extending our movement vocabulary, also provides us with one of the main 'tools' for observation, which Sherborne described as one of the most important aspects of her work. In her book, she says that:

> *... teachers of movement need to be aware of **what parts** of the body are moving, in **which direction** in space they are moving and, most important, **how** is the body moving?* (Sherborne, 2001, p. 55)*

A full study of Laban's work entails a vast undertaking over a period of time. However, due to its significance for Sherborne's work, a brief summary of his basic principles can be expressed in the following way (see also Figure 1.1).

All human activity, Laban believed, is the result of mental impulses to survive, to experience, to explore, to learn and to expand one's knowledge. These mental impulses are either the result of sensory experiences, which are fed in through the senses, or the result of life's experiences. These impulses have the same common result – movement – and the same common source – effort. 'Effort' is described by Laban as the common denominator for the various strivings of the body, and becomes observable as 'movement'. The quality of the resulting movement will depend on the inner attitude of the individual at the time of making the movement. The resulting movements will vary tremendously. Laban analysed movement in terms of what he called 'motion factors' and 'movement qualities'.

According to Laban, movements can be analysed into four motion factors:

1. Weight – strong or light
2. Space – direct or flexible
3. Time – fast or slow/sudden or sustained
4. Flow – bound or free.

```
        Motion factor                    Resulting movement quality
             |                                      |
          Weight                              Strong/Light
           Time                            Fast/Slow/Sudden
                                              or Sustained
Inner
Attitude to              EFFORT

          Space                              Direct/Flexible
           Flow                                Bound/Free
```

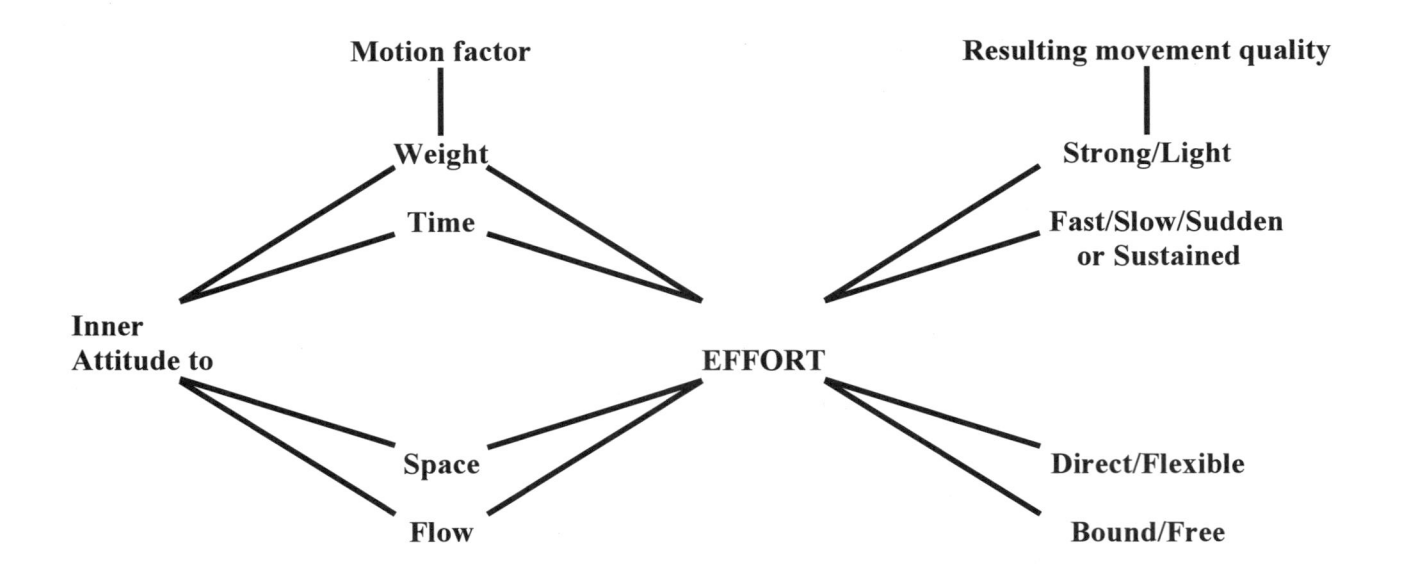

Figure 1.1 A simplified diagrammatic presentation of Laban's movement analysis

The initial two days, and the subsequent years, studying and latterly working with Laban were to become the overriding influence and inspiration for Sherborne's future work to the extent that she would often say, both in writing and conversation, that 'all I teach is based on Rudolf Laban's theory and analysis of movement'. An awareness of the basic principles of both Laban's movement analysis and Sherborne Developmental Movement (SDM) reveals how much Sherborne used Laban's work as the foundation for her own.

Following her time at the Art of Movement Studio, Sherborne returned to Bedford College of Education as a lecturer in Dance, and this was followed by a two-year period lecturing in the same subject at Bath Academy of Art. In 1950, Laban recommended that she should work with Gilbert and Irene Champernown at the Withymead Centre in Exeter as a visiting movement therapist. Here, she worked with people suffering from severe depressive illnesses, some of whom had suicidal tendencies. It was here, perhaps, that in drawing on her close association with Laban, who himself was intrinsically interested in the psychological impact of movement, she was to come to realisations which were to have a profound effect on her future work.

She continued to work in Exeter until 1965, a period spanning 15 years, but, as her work there did not continually fill her time, it was during these years that she entered the field of education, working as a tutor in Dance, Movement and Drama in several of the teacher training establishments in and around the Bristol area. At first, she worked with students and used her movement ideas 'to help the students to work together and to feel secure within the group using partner and group activities' (Sherborne, 2001),* and it would appear that the students began, almost by accident, to introduce the activities to the children they met in the course of their training.

So began for Sherborne, in the mid-1950s, the process of developing her ideas as a way of working with children with special needs. Drawing on the wealth of knowledge she had acquired from Laban, she recognised that, within his ideas about developing confidence in the body, an awareness of three-dimensional space, the confidence to explore relationships through movement, and an awareness of varying movement qualities as a tool for self-expression and creativity, there was a framework for her work with children with special needs. As her work evolved, she began to recognise the profound effect her work could have, not only on the children, but also on the people who were initiating the activities. The development of understanding, sensitivity, and mutual trust and confidence between everyone taking part in her movement experiences became an intrinsic part of her way of working.

Among the many tributes paid to Sherborne during the course of the 'Memorial Day of Celebration of her Work and Life' held in 1991, the following statements bear testimony to the value and high esteem in which her work is held, both in the UK and abroad.

> *I was always moved by Veronica's gentleness and her great ability as a communicator at all levels... My life has been much richer because I was lucky enough to work with her.* (UK)

> *I am writing to say how significant a contribution I think she made to special education.* (UK)

> *It is a language which can be used between many different professions.* (Norway)

> *I was deeply impressed by her personality, generosity and the beautiful way she gave her lessons.* (Norway)

> *We were deeply impressed by her as a person and teacher.* (Sweden)

> *Her work has had a profound effect on hundreds of teachers and children.* (Canada)

> *I am sure that I and many others who knew of Veronica's work couldn't help but admire her skill, knowledge and expertise – and be influenced by it.* (Australia)

Such was the impact of her work nationally and internationally.

In her memory, in recognition of her work, and also as a way of preventing it becoming fragmented in the future, Sherborne Associations have been set up in the UK, Belgium and Sweden, and there are many other countries, amongst which are Australia, Brazil, Canada, Eire, Finland, Germany, Italy, Japan, the Netherlands, Norway and Poland – the list continues to grow – where there is an on going interest in her work.

References
Hodgson, S. (1991) Unpublished 'flyer' for *London Drama*.
Laban, R. (1948) *Modern Educational Dance*. London: MacDonald and Evans.
Sherborne, V. (2001) *Developmental Movement for Children: Mainstream, special needs and pre-school* (2nd edn). London: Worth Publishing.
Thornton, S. (1971) *A Movement Perspective of Rudolf Laban*. London: MacDonald and Evans.

Websites
Sherborne Association UK: www.sherborne-association.org.uk

*Reprinted by kind permission of Worth Publishing from *Developmental Movement for Children* by Veronica Sherborne. 2nd Edition. Worth Publishing Limited 2001.

CHAPTER 2
The Evolving Theory:
Philosophical and Theoretical Aspects which Underpin Sherborne Developmental Movement

Through my experience of teaching and observing human movement, and of learning through trial and error, I have come to the conclusion that all children have two basic needs; they need to feel at home in their own bodies and so to gain body mastery, and they need to be able to form relationships. (Sherborne, 2001, p. xiii)*

This conclusion, drawn from her own personal and professional experiences and observation of her own children as they grew and developed, led Sherborne to establish two main objectives for her work, namely 'awareness of self' and 'awareness of others' – 'awareness of self' through the possibilities and capabilities of the whole body, or named body parts, in space; and 'awareness of others' through shared movement experiences (see Appendices 1 and 2). Drawing on her knowledge of child development, an intense interest in human movement and its psychological implications, and the knowledge and inspiration she acquired through her association with Rudolf Laban, she worked through the process of developing her unique approach, at first with children and young people with severe learning difficulties and, latterly, over a much broader spectrum of needs.

During the course of the intervening years between Sherborne's development of her approach and the present day, two very basic, but nonetheless fundamental, questions have emerged: firstly, 'What do we call Sherborne's work?'; and, secondly, 'How should we describe or define it?' When Sherborne herself was still practising and leading courses and workshops, we used to refer to the work as 'Sherborne' or simply 'Movement'. However, conversations with her on this particular subject were always very interesting and forthright, and about one thing she was quite firm. She would make it very clear that '*You* do not do Sherborne movement – *I* do my work in my way, and you take my ideas and use them in whatever way you feel is right for you – *you* create your own way of working.'

As early practitioners, this did not present a problem for us, but it did constitute a considerable dilemma in 1994 when we set up The Sherborne Association UK. Respecting her wishes that we did not refer to the work as 'Sherborne Movement', but at the same time wanting to retain its identity, it was decided in the first instance to call the work 'Developmental Movement – based on the work of Veronica Sherborne'. As this was rather long and cumbersome, it quickly became shortened to 'Developmental Movement'. Unfortunately, this in itself created confusion: 'What is Developmental Movement?' Is it the same as the Sherborne Movement we used to do?' So there was still some thinking to be done!

It was decided that The Sherborne Association, which had been set up in full consultation with Veronica's daughter, Sarah, should approach her and ask if we might reinstate the name in order to preserve the identity of her mother's work. Given the alternatives we had come up with, Sarah preferred the title by which the work is now known, 'Sherborne Developmental Movement' (SDM).

The question of the definition of the work is still very open-ended.
Again, Sherborne herself did not present us with a definitive description of her work, and maybe that was quite intentional on her part. She repeatedly made it very clear that her work was based on Rudolf Laban's principles and theory of human movement. This, in very simplified terms, focuses on self-exploration, and self-expression of responses to inner feelings and impulses, within an environment which is not bound by specifics and restrictive techniques. 'Definition', by interpretation, suggests boundaries, rules and limitations – quite an anathema to Laban's, and therefore, subsequently, to Sherborne's thinking.

Having said that, however, the question is one that is frequently asked, and it is helpful for new practitioners to have some form of definition of SDM on which to base their thinking or discourse. Sherborne herself was adamant that her work was *not* a therapy. 'I do not teach people to be therapists,' was the point she would make. However, there is no doubt in the minds of experienced practitioners that the work she developed, offered according to her guidance on implementation, does have *therapeutic qualities*.

Whilst not assuming to define SDM – it is still a topic encapsulated within discussions concerning the *evolving* theory – from my personal experience and understanding of Sherborne's work, I offer the following description:

> *Sherborne Developmental Movement (SDM) is a form of therapeutic intervention, which seeks to engage participants in interactive learning, through shared movement experiences which have their origins in the normal patterns of human development. These movement experiences are presented in an environment that is open to personal response, non-judgemental and firmly rooted within the concept of achievement and success.*

The purpose of this chapter is to explore and consider the evolving theory which underpins the practice and implementation of SDM. Before we proceed, however, there is a need to consider the term, 'evolving theory'.

In the Preface to the second edition of *Developmental Movement for Children* (2001), Sherborne's daughter, Sarah, describes her mother as a do-er rather than a writer. The format and content of Sherborne's text clearly follows her philosophy that a person has to 'experience' her work, and to '*do* my movements in order to fully understand them'. To her, practical participation in her movement experiences was her prime interest, and this is reflected in her text. The thrust of her writing is descriptive, with lateral references to the underlying theories as they became relevant within the context of her description. Apart from a chapter in which she focuses on 'Laban movement theory', which she always described as being the basis of her work, there is no definitive focus on the theoretical background to her work. However, careful study of her text reveals a profound understanding of and belief in the benefits derived from her way of working, in terms of its psychological and developmental implications.

It can be argued that there was not the need at the time of her writing (1990) for her to focus specifically on the theory behind her practice. However, at the present time, there is a clearly defined requirement for practitioners to have an awareness of the theoretical aspects of the work, and there is currently much deliberation surrounding the subject of the 'evolving theory'. Although in her time Sherborne presented her work as a personal movement programme, there is now the need to explore the theoretical background to her work.

As a result of many conversations shared with Sherborne, using her ideas in my own teaching, my role as a leader of workshops and courses on SDM, together with conversations and discussions with colleagues within the Sherborne Associations both in the UK and overseas, and through careful study of her texts, films and videos, I have had the opportunity to consider what I see as factors which contribute towards the philosophical and evolving theoretical framework underpinning Sherborne's way of working. It is those considerations, which I propose to outline here.

Since its conception in the late 1950s and early 1960s, Sherborne's work has continued to inspire workers in the fields of education, therapy and care to incorporate her ideas into their many and varied professional practices. What is it that makes the work so readily accessible and beneficial across such a broad spectrum of professions and needs? It is certainly not the complexity of the physical processes involved – on the contrary, the 'movements' in themselves are very simple in their application and are based on normal child development. Balancing, rolling, sliding, turning, twisting, walking, jumping and running – sometimes alone; at other times in shared movement experiences with another person or group of people – form the basis of her 'movement repertoire'. She described these basic movements in considerable detail in her book and supported her text with many carefully selected photographs.

For practitioners of SDM, it is imperative that readers take *Sherborne's* book as the definitive account of her way of working; for me to presume to restate that aspect of her work would be totally inappropriate. However, as a résumé of the basic principles of SDM, Appendix 1 shows, in diagrammatic form, the foundational aims and objectives of the work. Appendix 2 summarises the three categories of movement which form the basis of Sherborne's relationship work – 'caring or with' relationships, 'shared' relationships and 'against' relationships. I have also included, as Appendix 3, Stages 1–4 from the Sherborne Association document, 'Teaching Notes and Guidelines'. These stages show how some of the activities can be broken down and presented one step at a time, which not only allows for access at varying levels according to need and/or ability, but also can be used to demonstrate progress within the programme. This in itself, however, calls for a very strong word of warning. These stages are *not* intended to be used as a checklist to be worked through and ticked off. To use them in that way would be totally contrary to Sherborne's philosophy and way of working. It could well be that an individual may be working at varying stages for different movement experiences – this is highly likely.

That the movements she devised were simple and accessible, and did not require specific technical and physical skills in order to execute them, was totally intentional. It was not the movements in themselves that were the main focus of Sherborne's thinking. The way a child moves; how he[1] moves; his awareness of the surroundings; how he interacts with others; how a child *feels* about himself, and his concept of how others view him; how he reacts to others with whom he is sharing that time and space; how others react to him; the development of a positive self-image and a positive self-esteem; the building of trust and confidence in self and others – these ideas formed the absolute core of Sherborne's thinking, philosophy and practice.

The title of this chapter includes the word 'philosophy'. There is a need to clarify my understanding and intentional use of the word. When applying the word, the user has a clear definition *in his mind* as to what the word encapsulates, but to define it clearly can prove very difficult. Referring to selected dictionary definitions below, I find that 'philosophy' is:

> *The basic principles of a discipline. Any system of belief, values, or tenets.* (Collins English Dictionary, 1999)

> *A system of theories on the nature of things or of rules for the conduct of life.* (Oxford English Dictionary, 1949)

In the context of this chapter, I will be applying these two definitions, focusing particularly on the 'basic principles' of SDM as outlined in Sherborne's book (2001) and 'the rules for the conduct of life' in terms of the delivery and thinking which surrounds the implementation of SDM.

Through Sherborne's movement experiences, we are able to explore feelings and reactions which can contribute towards our assessment of self and others, and conversely their feelings towards us. The 'movements' are the vehicles by which such concepts are visited and explored, developed, accepted, rejected and rationalised. The activities are offered and taught in a way which is, most importantly, shared, enjoyable, fun and non-judgemental.

---

[1] It should be noted that the terms *he, his, him* refer to both male and female gender, and will continue to be used in this way throughout the book

Having suggested that it is not the 'movements' in themselves that are the most important aspect of Sherborne's work, we must now address the question, 'What is it, then, that contributes towards the quality and richness of the teaching and learning experience which SDM brings with it?' A carefully selected balance between movements that are developmentally appropriate, and the way those experiences are presented, are fundamental to the success of SDM sessions. Having selected 'appropriate' experiences, the pedagogy surrounding the successful implementation of SDM can be summarised in the old and very basic adage, 'It's not *what* you do; it's the way that you do it,' which prompted Sherborne to point out that: 'The quality of the interaction between the care-giver and the child has a profound effect on the child' (Sherborne, 2001).*

In the above quotation, Sherborne is speaking in the context of a 1:1 situation involving a carer and child, but the statement is equally applicable in any group session led or supported by two or more people. The essentials of the interaction between the group leader(s)/helpers and the participants are, in very simple terms:

- Showing the people we are working with that we **want** to be there with them
- Showing them that they are **valued** as individuals, and that their ideas and contributions to the session are also valued and respected
- Demonstrating that we view the session as a **shared experience**, in which everyone is equally involved and in which everyone's **efforts** are respected and celebrated, regardless of levels of achievement
- Ensuring that participants feel **emotionally safe and secure**.

Working in this way, SDM sessions become a very positive experience for everyone. The feeling of being valued and respected makes a significant contribution towards the development of self-confidence and a positive self-esteem, and the mutual respect and sensitivity towards others which are nurtured through this 'shared experience' can make a notable contribution towards the development of trust and confidence in self and in others.

Returning to the essentials of the interaction between group leaders and the participants, how can we show the people we are working with that we are working within such an ethos? What pedagogical principles do we need to apply in order to offer the maximum range of experiences and benefits to participants in an SDM session?

We want to be there
The teaching style we adopt at the beginning of a session will immediately convey messages of 'wanting to be part of the group'. Everyone taking off shoes and socks, the group leader(s) sitting on the floor and inviting the participants to do the same; the use of the word 'we' when talking about the session or the activities – all these actions indicate from the start that we wish to and intend to be part of the session. Our own body language and movements, our tone of voice, the way we address individuals should all reflect the ethos of the particular moment in the session. This will vary and change tremendously as the

session evolves, but, in changing, will communicate a total commitment to 'being there', and a flexibility which responds to the varying ambiences as they occur during the session.

Participants and their ideas are valued
Although the group leader(s) will have formulated a plan for the session, the movement activities will not be presented in a formal prescriptive way. Rather, ideas are presented to the group and participants asked to try out their own ways of doing things. If any new or innovative idea is noticed, then this should be shared and celebrated by the rest of the group, sometimes quite noisily with cheering and clapping and lots of praise!

Working in this way requires a flexible approach. Although the 'theme' of the session may be established (see Chapter 4), within that theme the movements undertaken might not follow a set plan, except perhaps when working with participants whose needs fall within the autistic spectrum, where it may be more appropriate to follow a set pattern. In the main, given the opportunity, participants in a movement session can become very creative, and, if this happens, then these innovative ideas must be applauded and shared. By making it apparent that we have noticed a particular individual's creativity, we make a notable contribution to that person's feeling of well-being and positive self-esteem. It is especially important that we look for such instances from the less out-going, more reticent participants, who in many other ways may not be noticed. Praising participants for their effort as well as for achieving specific goals is a fundamental aspect of SDM.

A shared experience
It is necessary for the session leader(s) to show that everyone in the group, including themselves, is equally involved. Again, the teaching style we adopt is crucial in this respect. In the first instance, it is important that we work at the same **level in space** as the participants. For example, if the group is exploring floor-based activities, then the group leader(s) should teach from floor level; if the group is 'sitting', then likewise the leader(s) should work from a sitting position. The same applies to movements when standing or moving around. If circumstances allow, during 'relationship' work, the group leader(s) should at times partner group participants – sometimes allowing them to take the initiative and to 'look after', 'roll' or work 'against' them. This is a very important aspect of Sherborne's thinking, as allowing the group participants to work with us on an equal basis indicates to them that we trust them just as much as we expect them to trust us – a big step in the development of mutual trust and respect.

Participants feel emotionally secure
It is important that we, at all times, offer reassurance to anyone in the group who may show signs of insecurity, nervousness or apprehension. There may be times when individuals are given permission not to participate in a particular experience, or times when the movement may be presented in a way which is more acceptable to them. For example, people who at first may not be able to tolerate 'being contained or cradled' as shown in Sherborne's book

(Sherborne, 2001, p.6, photograph no. 2) may prefer the more open type of support (Ibid., photograph no.3, p.7), or might simply be gently rocked from side to side with the supporter's hands just resting on their shoulders. It is also important that participants do not feel rushed and pushed into further activities. It is better to have a short movement session consisting of perhaps five or six movements, than a longer session during which a dozen or so activities have been rushed through. There must be plenty of time built in during which there are opportunities for personal interaction between the session leader and individual members of the group. This interaction may take the form of a simple touch on the hand or arm, a smile, a verbal remark or perhaps, more demonstratively, an arm around the shoulders.

The sensitive physical and empathetic support which participants receive during Sherborne's relationship work contributes tremendously towards the development of mutual trust and confidence that builds up between individuals and their carers or helpers. The important thing is that individuals do not feel threatened in any way and that they also feel physically and emotionally secure.

At the other end of the 'emotional' spectrum, Sherborne's 'against' relationship experiences (see Appendix 2) give us the opportunity to feel what it is like to be strong and assertive *without aggression.* In the past, on the subject of her 'against' relationship activities, Sherborne has been criticised for 'teaching children to fight'; therefore, it has been contended that children who already display aggressive tendencies should not take part in them. On the other hand, it can be argued that these are the very children, carefully managed in terms of 'partners', who should be involved in these particular experiences:

> *The aim of 'against' relationships is to help the child to focus and canalise energy and to develop determination. It is important for the child to discover and learn to control his or her strength in an appropriate way.*
> (Sherborne, 2001, p. 29)*

Perhaps it will be necessary, in the first instance, for a supporting adult to partner such individuals, and, when the participant does come to work with a peer, that the proceedings are carefully supervised and monitored.

Out of this discussion concerning the nature of the philosophy and evolving theory that underpins Sherborne's work, there emerges a number of key words and phrases which collectively summarise aspects of SDM that contribute towards its beneficial implementation.

In response to the question, 'Why does it work?', it can be said that SDM:

- Is based on **success** and **effort** – There is no prescribed way of doing the movements. The fact that there is no element of competition in Sherborne's work means that everyone taking part is able to succeed at his own level. 'Success' and 'effort' are celebrated and applauded, thus motivating the individual to move forward and strive for greater achievement.

- Is **differentiated** to accommodate a wide range of abilities, with activities ranging from very **simple** to **complex** movement experiences. For example, when working with participants who have multiple and severe disabilities, it is possible for them, with help and support from a more physically able person, to take part in many of Sherborne's movement activities and to share the experience even though they may not be able to become physically involved without help. On the other hand, many of Sherborne's activities require quite considerable skill in terms of balance, co-operation, and management of body weight, which offer challenges to more able participants.

- Offers a **positive experience** to all who take part, as everyone is able to succeed at his own level, and no-one feels threatened in any way.

- Is a **shared experience** – Everyone in the group is equally valued and involved, including the carers and group leader(s). Within a movement session, roles are often changed in that participants are encouraged, where appropriate, to 'look after' the caring person.

- Is based on the development of **trust** and **confidence** in self and others. Sherborne's relationship experiences allow participants to build up confidence in themselves in terms of their ability to look after another person and, conversely, to trust in the person who is working with them.

- Is **person-centred** – It is not prescriptive. Ideas are taken from individuals and developed within the group.

- Requires **flexibility** – Group participants are encouraged to explore ways of implementing the activities for themselves. Resulting ideas are taken from individuals and then shared and developed within the group.

- Encourages **creativity** – Often participants will produce activities which may not otherwise have been part of the session, thus extending the movement repertoire of the group. This feeling of creativity can also be instrumental in enhancing the positive self-esteem and self-image of the participants.

- Is based on the **observation** of reactions/skills/responses/movement preferences of the participants – The skills of being able to observe what is happening in the group, to read the reactions of the participants and to respond accordingly and effectively were considered by Sherborne to be necessary to facilitate a successful movement session.

- Is **enjoyable** and **fun**.

During the course of this chapter, we have discussed the formulation and ethos of SDM sessions. However, working in the way outlined above could beg the question, 'Where is the "progression" in SDM?' If everyone succeeds at their own level and sessions are based on existing abilities and preferences, how can group participants be expected to show any evidence of 'progress'?

In terms of the implementation of SDM, a constant factor throughout all movement experience is the continuing development of trust and confidence in self and others. With growing confidence comes the motivation to try out and experiment with new, perhaps more demanding, physical activities and to explore the possibility of developing a growing awareness in terms of relationships with others and our attitudes towards them.

SDM facilitates these progressions by providing, within its movement repertoire, a range of physical activities which, on the one hand, are very basic and simple to execute whilst, on the other, require considerable physical skills, which can lead very naturally into more formal gymnastics. In terms of a developing 'awareness of others', Sherborne's relationship activities can begin at the simplest 'meeting and greeting' level whilst we move around in the environment, but can also involve us in quite intricate and sensitive situations where our level of involvement and interaction with others require a considerable degree of interpersonal skills, social competence and emotional stability. Across this broad spectrum of involvement, there is the possibility for participants in SDM sessions to explore, achieve and, therefore, progress through being challenged and encouraged to take part in more demanding activities and situations. Any exploration of something 'new' demands a certain amount of risk-taking, but, as long as this 'exploration' is nurtured with sensitivity and respect, bearing in mind the key factors listed above, SDM offers the opportunity to explore, 'try out', and, with that, achieve progress in a supportive, non-judgemental atmosphere.

However, at the present time there *is* a need for exponents of Sherborne's work to have an understanding of 'Why we do what we do – why we do things in the way we do within the framework of Sherborne's movement experiences'.* As Janet Sparkes (in Sherborne, 2001) so rightly suggests in the preceding quotation, there is now the need to establish a consensus of recognised opinion about the 'evolving theory'. Much of what makes up the theoretical background of SDM now has to be teased out from conversations between Sherborne and practitioners who worked closely with her at the time, her many papers and, of course, from her definitive and only major text, *Developmental Movement for Children*. Those who were taught by her and were able to talk with her at some length were left in no doubt as to her personal conviction concerning the theory and philosophy which underpinned her practice.

It is also of great help to practitioners to have an awareness of the benefits of using Sherborne's approach. Again, although not specifically listed to any great extent in her book, Sherborne makes varying claims as to the 'benefits' of using her ideas and following her way of working. In terms of developing communication and language skills, she suggests that:

> *The children enjoy the play so much that learning the meaning of words comes easily as the action and the word are experienced together.* (Sherborne, 2001, p. 16)*

Discussing aspects of movement experiences, which incorporate balance, she says that:

> *It will be noticed that when children balance... they give their full attention to the activity. Attention spans can be increased if the motivation is strong enough.* (Ibid., p. 29)*

As part of the summary at the end of her book, listing ways in which Developmental Movement can help children, she includes amongst others that:

- *Children acquire a stronger sense of self...*
- *Children experience a sense of achievement...* (Ibid., p. 111)*

SDM encourages and recognises success within the capabilities of the individual. There are no prescriptive techniques or, moreover, a need to 'perform' the movement experiences. This is one of the keys to the success and benefit of using Sherborne's ideas in the way she advocated.

For the purposes of clarity, these beneficial effects can be summarised as contributing towards the development of:

- A positive self-esteem and self-image
- Self-confidence
- A positive sense of self
- Trust and confidence in self and others
- Altruism and sensitivity
- Positive aspects of 'relationships'
- Emotional security
- Creativity
- The opportunity for 'engagement' in a fun, relaxed, non-judgemental environment.

Developmentally, the use of Sherborne's approach allows for:

- Exploration of physical capabilities
- Coming to terms with physical limitations
- Exploration and the development of confidence to move out into space
- Development of concentration and attention skills
- Development of interpersonal skills
- An increase in social understanding and social interaction skills
- Broadening of communication skills.

It is very gratifying that many of these beneficial aspects are now being 'tested' by varying research projects (see Chapter 9) and results to date are very encouraging.

For those working in the field of education, SDM supports access to the National Curriculum across a broad band of core subjects whilst also providing a meaningful vehicle for inclusion.

Within these psychological and developmental benefits, using Sherborne's approach also offers many opportunities to explore social relationships and interaction, the notion of respect, both as in one individual's respect for 'another' and conversely the concept of how 'another respects me'. This two-way aspect of the work is of vital importance in the building of positive relationships and means of communication, verbal and non-verbal, between the individual and the carer/therapist/worker/teacher/parent, leading in no small way to an enhanced teaching/learning situation in whatever context it might occur.

Overall, the use of Sherborne's ideas in terms of experiences offered and the way those ideas are implemented, provides participants with the opportunity to explore and 'try out' many of life's experiences in a safe, supportive and non-judgemental environment.

It is important to recognise that when Sherborne devised her original repertoire of movement experiences she had 'a reason' for each of them – they were not activities decided upon at random. Through conversations with her, subsequent conversations with colleagues who also worked with her, and study of her texts and book, it is apparent that, when devising her movement experiences, she had the basic principles and objectives of her work – in terms of developing body awareness, spatial awareness, the trust and confidence to build positive relationships, and the ability to 'feel' creative' – firmly in her mind at all times. In psychological terms, the development of a positive self-image, self-esteem, self-concept and altruism were also fundamental to her thinking.

What was also of prime importance to her was an awareness of how children progress in the broad areas of physical, intellectual, emotional and social development. She would often say, and has written in her book, that she learnt a tremendous amount from simply watching her own children 'play'. The word 'play' was very significant to her, to the extent that, during the early years, she herself referred to her method as 'movement play', a term still used in some references to her work to this present day. However, as her ideas became more widely used, with adults with special needs as well as with children, she became aware that the term, 'play,' may not be entirely appropriate.

Whilst writing her book during the late 1980s and 1990, she became very concerned about a title for it, and I, and I am sure many others, had conversations with her about this! She finally decided upon 'Developmental Movement' for two main reasons – one being that 'developmental' reflected the fact that her movement experiences were based on the movements a child would normally make during his natural developmental processes – rolling, twisting, walking, running, jumping, curling, stretching, curling, balancing, etc. – as well as taking into account emotional and social developmental milestones; the other being that by incorporating the concept of 'development' she gave users of her ideas the licence to:

> ...*make use of the material described in this book in his or her own way. Teachers develop their own variations and ideas, as do the children they teach.* (Sherborne, 2001, p. 111)*

This broad spectrum of approach, and the way in which SDM is delivered, based on the individual needs and abilities of those to whom it is offered, are, in my opinion, the main reasons for its acceptance, use and successful implementation in so many differing professional practices. Those of us who are involved in the use of Sherborne's ideas in any way become part of an organic process. Providing the principles of the work are fundamentally rooted within the theoretical and philosophical framework which is presently addressed as the 'evolving theory', this process has within it the means to continue its development and progression across a broad spectrum of needs and environments.

References

Sherborne, V. (2001) *Developmental Movement for Children: Mainstream, special needs and pre-school* (2nd edn). London: Worth Publishing.

Sherborne Association (2002) 'Teaching notes and guidelines'. Available through The Sherborne Association UK (www.sherborne-association.org.uk).

*Reprinted by kind permission of Worth Publishing from *Developmental Movement for Children* by Veronica Sherborne. 2nd Edition. Worth Publishing Limited 2001.

CHAPTER 3
Psychological, Educational and Sociological Implications

In her book, Sherborne refers to her movements as 'experiences' pointing out very early on in her introduction that:

> *... the activities described in this book are referred to here as 'experiences' rather than 'exercises' because they combine both physical and psychological learning experiences.* (Sherborne, 2001, p. xiv)*

Throughout the book, she makes reference to the psychological effects her work can have, in terms of the development of personality and self-image, and the teaching and learning process. However, she makes no references to support and substantiate these claims. In order to understand this omission, there are several aspects which need to be considered.

Sherborne wrote from a position of total conviction, commitment and an absolute, life long belief in her work. In the 1970s, when she initially introduced her work into the field of special education, she (metaphorically speaking) 'placed her head in the jaws of the lion'! The responsibility for the education of children with severe and profound and multiple learning difficulties had recently moved from the health authorities to the local education authorities, where the education of these pupils was firmly grounded in the 'behaviourist/objectives model' – one very alien to her subjective, child-centred approach. She was continually challenged by other professionals as to the value, benefits and purpose of her way of working. However, she persisted in her work against the apparent odds and pressure, and perhaps it was this process which strengthened her personal resolve to maintain the integrity of her work and her absolute conviction as to its value. When she finally came to write her book, her prime interest was to record an account of *her* work, in a mainly descriptive style illustrated by photographs, which conveyed her total belief in what *she* was saying, without, as she saw it, the need for substantiating and supportive references.

To some extent, it can also be said that there was not the academic pressure to reference/substantiate/support writings, utterances and claims at the time of the initial publication of her book in 1990. Having said that, there is no doubt in my mind that she did have a broad insight into the possible psychological effects of her work. Her own work with Laban would have undoubtedly put considerable emphasis on the psychological effects of 'movement', whilst her personal library, which is, at the time of writing, held in trust by The Sherborne Association UK, contains copies of such books as *Children's Minds* (Donaldson, 1978), *Changing Children's Minds* (Sharron, 1987) and *The Psychology of Interpersonal Behaviour* (Argyle, 1983), among many others. However, things have changed considerably in the intervening years between the initial publication of her book in 1990 and the publication of the second edition in 2001, and now it can be argued that there is a need for her work to be referenced and substantiated if it is to be viewed and valued to its full potential and merit.

We do not know for sure whose or which psychological theories Sherborne had in mind when she referred to her 'psychological experiences'. It was not within her personal remit at the time of writing her book to reveal that; therefore it is up to us, the present-day practitioners, to surmise that. This requires reading around publications based on the work of influential and respected theorists – psychologists, sociologists and educational researchers, past and present – and then, with a knowledge and awareness of Sherborne's work as she has presented it in her book, identifying references which support her claims of her work's benefits.

From my own reading in preparation for this chapter, I have selected what can be only a very small proportion of the material available which can be seen to support and substantiate Sherborne's work. I have selected findings and theories which I find particularly relevant and which, in my view, although they may refer to a very different context, do conceptualise the theory and philosophy which underpin Sherborne Developmental Movement (SDM). My intention in this chapter is to cross-reference Sherborne's thinking and the 'evolving theory' outlined in Chapters 1 and 2 with that of investigators and researchers past and present who contribute towards the current consensus of educational, psychological and sociological thinking.

Philosophical Considerations and Teaching and Learning Styles

> *Learning is a life long adventure. It's a never-ending voyage of exploration to create your own personal understanding.* (Rose and Nicholl, 1997, p. 3)

Education is a life long process. It is certainly not confined to the years spent in school and further education. Education and learning, in the broadest sense, involve changes in behaviour, knowledge base and attitude. It goes without saying that the attitudes and philosophical beliefs of those of us who impart knowledge, share experiences or are 'changing behaviour' within the context of Sherborne's work, as in any other situation, will be reflected in the behaviour we adopt as facilitators during SDM sessions. Discussing the philosophy of the educator in terms of delivery, Peter Arnold, in *Education, Movement and the Curriculum*, maintains that:

> *It is [the]...respect of one person for another that should form a constituent part of all educative situations.* (Arnold, 1988, p. 3)

In the context of SDM, it is exactly the same philosophy which applies. As explained in Chapter 2, the focus of Sherborne's thinking was not the movements themselves, although they were designed with specific aims in mind (see also Chapters 1 and 2 in Sherborne (2001)); it was the developing awareness of self and the interaction between the participants. She was not interested in skill levels and performance as such, but in the positive concepts which participants acquired about themselves and others by participating in her movement experiences. The responsibility for conveying those positive concepts she saw as being very much in the hands of the people who were leading the movement sessions, in that (to expand upon the quote used earlier):

> *The quality of the interaction between the care-giver and the child has a profound effect on the child... [The] child should experience success, a sense of achievement, and an awareness of self worth.* (Sherborne, 2001, pp. 3–4)*

This quality of interaction will depend on the 'messages' that we, as facilitators of an SDM session, give out to the participants. As discussed in the previous chapter, the successful communication of these messages will depend very much on the attitude and teaching style we adopt whilst running our SDM sessions.

Although presented in a very different context, the thinking which surrounds Feuerstein's Instrumental Enrichment Programme, based on mediated learning experiences as described by Sharron in *Changing Children's Minds*, relates very closely to the positive, personal interactions between the teacher and the pupil as advocated in SDM. Feuerstein, in his mediated learning experiences, was concerned mainly with solving intellectual problems, but his philosophical and theoretical arguments concerning ways to motivate the child towards developing those skills are also implicit within the teaching styles which accompany the implementation of SDM.

Sharron, describing one of the objectives of Instrumental Enrichment, says it is:

> *...to change children's images of themselves as passive receivers... to actively creative masters and generators of information... It is the task of teacher to produce the awareness in the learner of his or her contribution in the solution of a given problem... This awareness can become a source of knowledge about one's own ability to affect the world... and may lead to a greater readiness to accept responsibilities.* (Sharron, 1994, p. 104)

Taught from a similar philosophy, SDM can make a very positive contribution towards developing the awareness to which Sharron refers.

In the previous chapter, we discussed at some length the 'teaching styles' we need to adopt if SDM is to be implemented successfully. Discussing teaching styles in general terms, it can be said that in any teaching/learning situation the teaching style we adopt will immediately convey the ethos of the intended interaction between the teacher and the learner. In some cases, the interaction is very formalised, with the teacher intent on 'delivery' and the pupils 'receiving'; in some, there is a mixture of 'delivery and dialogue'; whilst in other circumstances, the process is viewed as a 'shared experience'. All teaching styles have their appropriateness according to the aims of the interaction between the teacher and the learner. In SDM, the teaching style most frequently adopted, due to the nature of the work, has to fall into the third category of those briefly outlined above.

Success
With reference to the key word, 'success' (see previous chapter), Feuerstein reflects that:

> ... a child's success at solving intellectual problems... is as dependent on the feelings of competence, as on his actual competence, for if the first is not present children become so convinced of their likely failure that they do not attempt to solve problems... (Ibid., 1994, p. 46)

Furthermore:

> ... the excitement of success that is conveyed by parents [include also teachers, carers, therapists, etc.]... when they are mediating competence to their children, provokes a need in the children to seek goals for themselves and to try to reach those goals. (Ibid., p. 48)

Included in *Changing Children's Minds* is an account of the work of Professor Klein, who has extended the application of Feuerstein's theories into the field of early childhood development in terms of an early intervention programme referred to as the More Intelligent Sensitive Child (MISC) programme. This programme has:

> ...particular relevance for its potential to prevent problems... including the lack of parent child attachment, poor emotional development and the lack of the development of prosocial skills. (Coulter in Sharron, 1994, p. 354)

Recent modifications (1992) to the MISC programme have broadened it out considerably to include 'feelings, excitement and empathy'. A significant inclusion in terms of SDM is the focus on:

> ... the critical nature of reciprocity, turn-taking and following children's initiatives as well as focusing on adult initiated interactions. (Ibid., p. 357)

As this is put forward as a later modification to the work of Klien and Hundeide, we cannot take this as an example of support for Sherborne's work, but, interestingly, rather as an example of how her thinking is being paralleled and substantiated in recent times.

The books, *Accelerated Learning* (Rose, 1996) and the subsequent *Accelerated Learning for the 21st Century* (Rose and Nicholl, 1997), put forward some very forceful arguments for a far more creative approach to learning. It is interesting to note how Rose points out that:

> ...since **non-verbal communication** is a right brain activity and non-verbal actions account for perhaps **80% of all communication** we can see just how much our left brain orientated learning systems may be starving our intellectual development. (Rose, 1996, p. 16)

Rose is concerned with the education of children in the mainstream setting. Much of the argument concerning the methods by which children are taught at the present time, and the ways in which he (and, latterly, he and Nicholl), advocate education should be happening, are in total accord with the teaching/learning styles and processes encapsulated within SDM, where much of the communication is non-verbal and 'creativity' is encouraged at all times.

Accelerated Learning, which focuses on a dynamic, creative approach to learning, has evolved out of the work of Dr Georgi Lozanov, Bulgaria's leading research psychologist. Rose, reflecting on attending a class using the 'Lozanov method' remarks that it was:

> ...noticeable that every single element of the class is positive. No criticism. Just encouragement... Everything is focused to ensure effective, stress free learning. (Ibid., p. 91)

As already pointed out in Chapter 2, SDM is a 'positive' experience, built on success. Continuing the theme of 'success', summarising *Accelerated Learning*, Rose advocates that:

> ...suggestion can improve actual performance greatly – not by creating new abilities but by unblocking the negative suggestion that something cannot be done.

Furthermore:

> ...creating a belief in success and a positive self-image, will, when allied to a sound and realistic learning programme, create great success. (Ibid., p. 168)

The notion of 'success' is further pursued by Rose and Nicholl (1997) when they focus on the all important 'culture of success' which includes:

- *No put downs **ever**. Look for every opportunity to show how everyone is smart, albeit in different ways.*
- *Teach students to encourage each other... Look for ways they can work as a team so everyone's success matters to the others.* (Rose and Nicholl, 1997, p. 294)

Reference to the key words listed in Chapter 2 shows how closely this philosophy relates to Sherborne's way of working.

Finally, in terms of teaching styles and the links between SDM and Accelerated Learning, another of the aspects of SDM highlighted in the key words in the previous chapter is that SDM is 'non-prescriptive' – there is no right or wrong way of 'doing' the activities, and participants are encouraged to 'think of ways for themselves'. Likewise, in Accelerated Learning, creative thinking is encouraged at all times and:

> ...it is important to stress that most of the time you are looking for 'an' answer, not 'the' answer. (Ibid., p. 292)

Creativity
The theme of 'creativity' 'which represents an ability to generate novel ideas in innovative solutions, which are appropriate in context and valued by others' (Shaffer, 1996), is also very much part of Sherborne's work (see previous chapter). Participants of SDM sessions are encouraged at all times to think of different ways of doing the movements for themselves. Having our creativity acknowledged and recognised by others provides a tremendous boost for our self-esteem and feeling of being 'valued and respected'.

Discussing the competitive aspects of games, Arnold maintains that:

> ...the emphasis... is not on the end result – winning or loosing – but rather on what takes place and the manner in which it takes place. (Arnold, 1988, p. 64)

This can also be applied to Sherborne's notion that there is no element of competition in her work; it was the manner in which individuals participated that was her main concern. Arnold goes on to say that:

> ...the teacher's most important role in getting the children to be creative and expressive is the establishment of an encouraging, stimulating, yet secure atmosphere. (Ibid., p. 99)

Arguing from a much broader perspective, Rose and Nicholl suggest that:

> ...learning to think logically and creatively is critical if we are to solve complex personal and social problems effectively. (Rose and Nicholl, 1997, p. 17)

Accepting that they were arguing from a much broader platform which encompasses elements from across the national education system, their ideas, nevertheless, support the theory behind Sherborne's 'relationship' activities, which encourages us to explore the notion of developing positive relationships built on a basis of mutual trust and confidence, in an exploratory, non-threatening and creative way.

The Role of 'Emotion' within the Learning Process

As previously discussed, feeling secure and confident, not only in our own body and self-image, but also in our contacts and dealings with the people with whom we are working, is fundamental to SDM if it is to generate its full impact. It is the 'messages' we, as supporters, convey to the people we are working with, through the attitudes and teaching styles we adopt, which will provide the basis on which this confidence and feeling of emotional security will depend and upon which Sherborne places so much importance. The sense of its importance is shared by Feuerstein, as crucial to the success of his Instrumental Enrichment Programme. Discussing 'sharing behaviour', it is pointed out that:

> ...because of its highly charged emotional quality, sharing behaviour ensures the effectiveness of the mediator in other adult–child interactions. (Sharron, 1994, p. 49)

Furthermore, Feuerstein's theory has contained within it:

> ...many complex elements which are of great relevance to theorists and practitioners in a variety of fields and settings. Some of these elements include an intense focus on... the potential for having a great empowering effect on caregivers through the understanding of the importance of their relationship with their children. (Ibid., p. 351)

This is very relevant to SDM, in which the essence of the work is the quality of the interaction between everyone taking part in the session, be they participants, session leaders or supporters/helpers.

Rose and Nicholl have some very powerful things to say about the importance of emotion within the teaching and learning situation. They argue that if you:

> ...deliberately involve the emotions, you harness powerful forces that make learning much more effective. (Rose and Nicholl, 1997, p. 51)

As in SDM, alongside this feeling of emotional security, there also needs to be a sense of 'fun'. Learning must be exciting, successful and enjoyable, and we can instigate this by:

> ...ensuring that learning is emotionally positive... it generally is when... there is humour and encouragement...and enthusiastic support. (Ibid., 1997)

Summarising the importance of 'emotion' within the learning process, MacCoby and Martin suggest that:

> ...the emotional context of an experience profoundly affects the way in which it is remembered and has a bearing on current functioning. (MacCoby and Martin, cited in Dunn, 1992, p. 81)

This is a notion which is also supported by Rose and Nicholl, who point out that:

> ...we know emotion is very important in the educative process because it drives attention, which drives learning and memory. (Rose and Nicholl, 1997, p. 51)

Sherborne stresses the importance of 'emotional security' very early on in her book, where she writes that:

> When the child finds he or she can trust a partner to physically support, contain and handle him or her in a trustworthy way, that child develops not only physical confidence but also a sense of being emotionally secure. (Sherborne, 2001, p. 4)*

The Development of Concentration and Attention Skills
Attention and concentration are essential elements in any learning process. Sherborne recognised this, and stated of her 'against' relationship activities:

> ...if children learn to use their strength in a focused way, especially along direct, linear pathways, they will develop skills in attending, in directing their energy and concentrating on a job. (Ibid., pp. 30–31)*

Shaffer (1996) in *Developmental Psychology* gives considerable space to the subject of 'attention', arguing that:

> ...there is nothing we consciously do that is not influenced by the interpretation of the world around us...perception is at the heart of human development... (p. 240) ...perceptual development in childhood is largely a matter of the development of attention (p. 228) ...as children's attention spans increase they are better able to plan what they are to attend to and to ignore distractions. (p. 307)

This view is supported by Feuerstein (cited in Sharron, 1994), who suggests that 'crucial to a child's cognitive development is the need to be able to focus perception and attention'.

One of the theoretical aspects of Sherborne's 'against' relationship activities is that, in requiring us to focus and concentrate our energy 'against' that of our partner, we actually 'feel' what it is like to concentrate and focus our attention on the task in hand. Chapter 9 of this book outlines a classroom-based, action research project in which Sherborne's claim that her work can contribute to the development of concentration and attention skills was put to the test. The results were very gratifying in that the incidents of concentrating and attending behaviour did show an increase following an SDM session. (The same research project also looked into the numerical incidence of positive social interaction following an SDM session.)

The Sense of Self, a Positive Self-Esteem and Altruism

How we interact with others is greatly influenced by how we feel about ourselves, how we perceive what others think of us, and *our* attitudes and feelings towards others. The two prime aims of Sherborne's work, '**awareness of self**' and '**awareness of others**', address precisely these major factors in personal development. The development of a positive self-esteem and sensitivity towards the feelings of others is fundamental throughout all her 'movement experiences', and we have already discussed at some considerable length how SDM can make a very positive contribution towards the acquisition of these attributes. The major importance that Sherborne attached to the way her work was implemented in order for this to happen is well supported by aspects of 'psychological thinking'.

Shaffer, discussing 'self-esteem', tells us that recent research findings suggest a consensus of thinking that:

> *... both self knowledge and self esteem may depend to a large extent on the way others perceive and react to our behaviour.* (Shaffer, 1996, p. 470)

He adds that children who are in an environment where:

> *...they receive praise for their successes and are not over criticized for 'an occasional failure' are more likely to seek challenges and display high levels of achievement motivation.* (Ibid. p. 477)

In the book, *Growing Up in a Changing Society* (Woodhead et al., 1991), there are several references to the role of the teacher in the acquisition of a sense of self, including:

> *Children acquire an awareness of 'self' through interaction with others; via their attitudes and values, rewards and punishments.* (Woodhead et al., 1991, p. 156)

Accepting the findings of research (Nash, 1973) that children behave according to the perception they have of how their teachers perceive them, it therefore follows that:

> *... the teacher... has a powerful role to play in the child's acquisition of 'self image'.* (Crocker and Cheeseman, cited Ibid., p. 156)

A positive self-esteem and a feeling of self-worth, without arrogance, have a profound effect on how we feel about others. Personal insecurities will be reflected in our attitude towards the personalities and behaviours of others. 'Confidence in self' will allow us to view others from a much broader, sympathetic and generous perspective. To be able to view the world totally from another's point of view is a gift with which, in its entirety, very few of us have been endowed. Having said that, however, I would venture to say that there are also very few of us who do not have any feelings at all towards our companions, in whatever context or relationships we find ourselves. The possible exception to that rule may be found in children with autistic spectrum disorders (ASDs). Although not strictly within the context of this chapter, it is worth noting that there are several case histories which indicate the success of SDM in this field.

Sherborne's 'relationship' work concentrates on the development of a positive attitude and a growing sensitivity and sensibility towards the people we are working with – attributes which, it is hoped, will then be generalised into everyday life experiences.

The feeling of altruism – which dictionaries define as 'concern for the welfare of others…selflessness' and 'regard for others as a principle of action' – is embodied in Sherborne's second prime objective, 'awareness of others'. Shaffer defines what he terms the development of the pro-social self as:

> *… the selfless concern for the welfare of others that is expressed through pro-social acts such as sharing, co-operating and helping.* (Shaffer, 1996, p. 559)

According to Shaffer, these pro-social acts are not possible without a degree of social cognitive development which brings with it the ability to role-take from another person's perspective.

We have to understand and appreciate what and how the other person is feeling before we are in a position to empathise with the way in which they are dealing with a given situation. The process needed in order to be able to view a situation in an altruistic way is, firstly, to be in a position to understand in realistic terms the nature of the other person's feelings/attitudes, and then to be able to imagine how we would feel in similar circumstances. Shaffer sees the ability to 'role play' as being developed through:

> *… equal status contacts with friends and peers [which] are crucial to social cognitive development. They contribute indirectly by fostering growth of role-taking skills and directly by providing the experiences children need to learn what others are like.* (Ibid., p. 501)

Although his book was written some years after Sherborne was developing her ideas, his words, as a way of substantiating her work, could not have been more supportive. One way of reinforcing altruism, he suggests, is by:

> *… structuring play activities so that children are likely to discover the benefits of co-operating and helping one another.* (Ibid., p. 566)

He asks if it is possible to promote altruism by persuading young people to think of themselves as generous or helpful individuals. He answers this question by pointing out that research suggests that positive verbal reinforcement of 'nice' or 'helpful' acts promotes empathy and altruism. He goes on to say that:

> *...encouraging youngsters to think of themselves as altruistic is one way to promote acts of kindness.* (Ibid., p. 565)

> *Children and adolescents who receive training to further role-taking skills... subsequently become more charitable, more co-operative and more concerned about the needs of others.* (Ibid., p. 561)

Every aspect of the above three quotations can be directly cross-referenced to Sherborne's work, in which participants are continually being encouraged to respect the feelings of others, to develop a sensitivity to their needs, to work co-operatively together and to focus on 'helping one another'. Sherborne's second prime objective, 'awareness of others', implemented by way of her 'relationship' activities, allows us to 'practise' and develop a concept of these very important 'socially interactive life skills' in a practical and supportive environment.

The Process of Development within the Social Context

Running parallel to the development of 'awareness of others', there is also the prime objective of Sherborne's work, 'awareness of self', which focuses on 'personal development'. No matter which aspect of SDM we are concentrating on at any given time, the process takes place within a social context, either through experiences shared with one other person or within a group of people. In recent years, the consensus of psychological thinking and debate concerning child development has shifted somewhat from the formalised, classical, psychological 'testing and investigation' to investigations which take into account the cultural and social context in which the child is growing up. Having said that, however, it is not possible to discuss the subject of 'child development' without reference to the work of Piaget. It is the circumstances that surrounded his work which are of particular interest, and which lead us on, through reference to contemporary work, to links with SDM.

The general outcomes of Piaget's work led him to refer to 'the lone child as an experimenter':

> *Teaching may have a place... but what is learned is ultimately dependent on what children are able to assimilate to their emerging mental schemas.* (Piaget, 1965, cited in Woodhead and Light, 1991, p. 51).

Less influential until more recent times, but running parallel with Piaget, is the work of Vygotsky, who coincidentally was also born in 1896, but who died at the early age of 40 years. Vygotsky, unlike Piaget, focused his attention on 'the child in the cultural and social context' and the role of the 'supporting adult' in the developmental process. As a point of interest, it is worth noting that Piaget and Vygotsky reflect in their respective theories their own cultural influences. Piaget's 'lone child as an experimenter' reflects Western individualism, whereas Vygotsky's 'child in a social context' reflects the collective system of the, then, USSR.

That Piaget's findings and conclusions continue to have considerable influence cannot be denied. However, his work has subsequently been scrutinised and often challenged. Margaret Donaldson, in her book, *Children's Minds* (1978), advocates the moving of the study of child development away from the classical, clinical setting, towards a more cultural, social environment, in which tasks are presented in a way that makes 'greater human sense'.

The intrinsic nature of SDM dictates that it is 'development within the social context' which can be directly correlated with Sherborne's work, in which the role of the supporting adult and the quality of the interaction is of vital importance. For this reason, the final section of this chapter will focus on the work of Vygotsky, the ideas which have developed out of his work, and the work of Judy Dunn as outlined in her book, *The Beginnings of Social Understanding* (1992).

Discussing Vygotsky's thinking, Woodhead and Light (1991) describe the process of child development as a constructive one but state:

> *...it is not the child alone who is doing the constructing. Rather, the construction of knowledge and understanding in development is conceived as a fundamentally social activity.* (Ibid., p. 61)

> *...processes that go on 'between' the child and others become the basis for processes which subsequently go on 'within' the child.* (Ibid., p. 60)

A phrase seminal to Vygotsky's work is his 'zone of proximal development' which:

> *...provides a... central and constructive role for the adults fostering the child's development.* (Ibid., p. 61)

This is seen by Tharp and Gallimore as:

> *...a multitude of 'growing edges', which relates to all areas of developing competence,* (Ibid., p. 61)

and which is nurtured and encouraged to develop. Vygotsky maintained that self-supported competence might be achieved only after successful performance had been established subsequent to 'assisted learning'.

Out of Vygotsky's 'zone of proximal development' evolved Bruner's theory of 'scaffolding', in which:

> *...the role of the adult... is to lend support to the child's own constructive activity, enabling the child to achieve the requisite skill or understanding, and then remove progressively the support in such a way that the child can function autonomously.* (Ibid., p. 61)

This concept is entirely in keeping with Sherborne's 'levels of support', which she sees basically as being broken down into three stages. During the course of involvement in SDM sessions the participants are:

1. Supported by a more physically able, more competent adult/person
2. Encouraged, where appropriate, to be 'in charge' or to 'look after' their supporting partner
3. Encouraged to work with 'peer group' partners and to devise their own ways of implementing the movement activities.

The Beginnings of Social Understanding is an account of Judy Dunn's research into the development of social understanding of children, mainly in their second and third years, within the family setting. However, there is much which she says that can be directly linked to the philosophy and theory which underpins Sherborne's work, with the proviso that we are often working with people who may be experiencing developmental delay in one or several aspects of their developmental pattern, and there are many cases in which such interpersonal skills need to be practised and developed beyond her young infant age range. In general terms she maintains that:

> *... it is important for [children] to begin to understand the intentions, feelings and actions of others who share their world and to comprehend the social rules of that world.* (Dunn, 1992, p. 1)

> *... children develop their powers of communication, understanding and thought, their emotional security and their sense of themselves within a complex social framework.* (Ibid., p. 3)

> *... to become a person... children must develop powers of recognizing and sharing emotional states, of interpreting and anticipating others' reactions ... [and] of understanding the relationships between others.* (Ibid., p. 5)

Her research suggests that role reversal is part of natural development at an early age. She observed that:

> *...there were sequences of play in which the children not only took one role in a joint game, but were able to reverse roles... [The] smoothness with which two year olds carried out such role reversals illustrates how they could anticipate the actions of the other and co-ordinate their own behaviour.* (Ibid., pp. 115–116)

She also noted that by the second year:

> *... children respond empathetically to the distress of others, and they are interested in the 'feeling state' of others... [They] develop increasing sensitivity to the goals and intentions of others, a sensitivity that is evident in conflict and in their helpful and co-operative behaviour.* (Ibid., p. 170)

Being effective in such matters as getting co-operation and attention, providing comfort for someone who is in distress, Dunn suggests, greatly influences children's feelings about themselves, but this entails:

> *... monitoring the response of others to oneself, their approval or disapproval, pleasure or displeasure.* (Ibid., p. 178)

Our work with SDM, in which we are encouraged to become aware of the feelings of others, gives us many opportunities to practise the life skills to which Dunn refers in a supportive, reciprocal environment.

It has been my direct intention in this chapter to make reference to published works, which, in my view, substantiate and support Sherborne's decision to refer to her movements as 'movement experiences'. As we have already discussed in Chapter 2, Sherborne's 'movement experiences' are, in the main, straightforward and simple, requiring no great technical skill or physical ability to execute. That '...there is no competitive element in the movement experiences...' (Sherborne, 2001)* and that effort and success, as a result of meaningful participation, is shared and celebrated makes participation in an SDM session a very positive experience. If all the educational, psychological and sociological benefits discussed in Chapter 2, and subsequently substantiated in this chapter, are to come to fruition then it is essential that those of us who offer SDM sessions give ourselves time to internalise the essentials which this very enriching way of working has to offer. This cannot happen overnight. We have to give ourselves and the people we are working with time to assimilate the 'feel' and impact of Sherborne's work. She insisted that we need to *do* the movements for ourselves in order to understand their full potential and benefits. The confidence of *all* of us taking part in SDM increases as we run our sessions as a 'shared experience' in which we grow together.

The need for this sequence, the way we offer SDM sessions in practical terms and taking into account necessary 'levels of support' with varying groups and issues we may encounter along the way will be the focus of Chapter 4.

References

Argyle, M. (1983) *The Psychology of Interpersonal Behaviour*. London: Penguin.

Arnold, P.J. (1988) *Education, Movement and the Curriculum*. Lewes: Falmer.

Donaldson, M. (1978) *Children's Minds*. London: Fontana.

Dunn, J. (1992) *The Beginnings of Social Understanding*. Oxford: Blackwell.

Coulter, M. (1994) 'New directions and applications'. In H. Sharron (1994) *Changing Children's Minds*. Birmingham: The Sharron Publishing Company.

Nash, R. (1973) *Classrooms Observed: The teacher's perceptions and the pupil's performance*. London: Routledge and Kegan Paul.

Rose, C. (1996) *Accelerated Learning*. Aylesbury: Accelerated Learning Systems Ltd.

Rose, C. and Nicholls, M.J. (1997) *Accelerated Learning for the 21st Century*. London: Piatkus.

Shaffer, D.R. (1996) *Developmental Psychology: Childhood and adolescence* (4th edn). Pacific Grove: Brooks/Cole Publishing.

Sharron, H. (1994) *Changing Children's Minds*. Birmingham: The Sharron Publishing Company.

Sherborne, V. (2001) *Developmental Movement for Children: Mainstream, special needs and pre-school* (2nd edn). London: Worth Publishing.

Woodhead, M., Light, P. and Carr, R. (eds) (1991) *Growing Up in a Changing Society*. Milton Keynes: The Open University.

Woodhead, M. and Light, P. (1991) *Child Development in a Social Context*. Milton Keynes: The Open University.

*Reprinted by kind permission of Worth Publishing from *Developmental Movement for Children* by Veronica Sherborne.
2nd Edition. Worth Publishing Limited 2001.

PART 2

From Theory into Practice

CHAPTER 4
Practical Aspects of a Sherborne Developmental Movement Session

In this 'practical' chapter, we will be thinking about a number of factors that need to be taken into account when running a Sherborne Developmental Movement (SDM) session, which should help towards a successful movement outcome, for both the session leaders and the participants. These factors include observation and assessment, communication, the content and length of a session, how to start and finish a session, and safety. Within the issue of 'safety', we will also consider 'lifting' and 'touch'. The latter part of the chapter will look into how we use SDM with individuals or groups with varying types of abilities and needs.

Observation and Assessment
Knowledge of the Participants – Assessment of Skills and Abilities
Before we begin our movement sessions, we need to have an awareness of the participants' abilities and needs. Whether they are ambulant, need 1:1 support, can function in a group situation, can tolerate physical contact or need the additional support of basic equipment such as blankets, are all factors which need to be taken into account. The needs and abilities of individuals may vary within the group, and these must be catered for before the sessions begin. There is nothing worse than losing the continuity of a movement session because you do not have that extra support on hand.

In our assessment, it is important that we look at the positive aspects of each individual and use their existing skills to fulfil or compensate for their particular needs. The assessment gives the baseline from which we work and acts as a benchmark for future comparisons. It is also essential to acknowledge changes which may occur as a result of progression or regression, and to reflect that in future sessions. As the movement is based on physical and interactive involvement, recorded observation is a very important part of the assessment strategy, and also forms part of the ongoing assessment. Appendix 4 consists of an assessment procedure, compiled by the author and George Hill, which can be used in this capacity.

Recording of Current Performance – Written and Video
In order to progress the movement in a meaningful way for each participant, it is essential that there should be ongoing assessment. Ideally, each session should be recorded either in writing or by use of video, but realistically this may not be possible. Video is the most effective and efficient way of recording, but this is very demanding on available resources as, in the first place, you need someone to do the videoing. This might well take someone who could otherwise be giving support during the session.

If it is not possible to record each session, then it is important to record any noticeable changes in terms of body or spatial awareness or response to relationship work, as these are important aspects of Sherborne's work. It is also important to make a note of any incident of individuality or creativity which might have occurred. Videoing a session at regular intervals of, say, every three months will give a good overall impression of how the sessions are progressing or otherwise, or where additional emphasis might be needed.

Communication
Reacting to Vocalisation and Verbal Language Responses
Movement offers a very positive opportunity for the use of language at all levels. It is very easy to do things inadvertently for people who are not able to communicate verbally, without allowing them the opportunity to make their feelings known. This is especially so in a movement session where the activity is transient, and responses may go unnoticed. It is necessary, as far as possible, for us to learn the intended communication of particular vocalisations used by individuals who are unable to communicate verbally. They often have very explicit meanings, are usually made in response to specific actions, and carry explicit communication of such feelings as pleasure, anxiety, frustration, tiredness or happiness in response to the varying movement experiences we offer them. It is also important that we talk to participants – telling them what is about to happen, reassuring them if necessary, and, where possible, eliciting a vocal response. This should also be the case, of course, with participants who are able to verbalise. It is important that, at all times, they are encouraged to reflect on what is happening during the session, in terms of their feelings, preferences and ambivalences! In this respect, where appropriate, participants should also be encouraged to say why they feel the way they do. Communication *at all levels* is an intrinsic part of SDM.

Recognising and Reacting to Body Language
Body language is as important in some instances as verbal language. It requires a lot of skill to disguise or hide body language, and, for the participants who have no verbal language, it is an essential means of communicating. As with vocalisations, we need to develop the skill of recognising body language, particularly when we are working with people who have profound and multiple difficulties. With their bodily reactions, the participants will indicate what effect the movement is having for them. A grimace, a smile, an eye, head, hand, finger or limb movement are all very significant. Showing recognition of these signs and subsequently responding to them will, in the first place, indicate to the participants that we are aware of their feelings, and, subsequently, guide the direction in which the movement will go.

Body language can also communicate our overall demeanour in more general ways. Sherborne used to pay particular attention to the hands and feet of a person lying on their backs 'relaxing'. 'People who are relaxed,' she would say, 'will allow their feet to fall out to the side, and will lie with the palms of their hands facing upwards.' A tense, nervous person, when lying on the floor, will be reluctant to let his head rest. He will keep lifting it and looking around so that he can see what is going on. In very general terms, the body of a tense person will not be able to give in to 'free-flow' movements; the body will be in a constant 'bound' state. We need to be aware of this involuntary type of communication and respond to it with appropriate movement experiences which will allow participants to experience 'opposite' movement qualities.

Positive Communication
All communication with the participants should be positive. The essence of SDM is that it is a positive experience for all concerned. All levels of achievement, effort and involvement should be acknowledged with words of praise and encouragement to strive for further success. If the activity does not fall within the intended outcomes, it is not a case of saying it is wrong, but saying rather, 'That was a good try. Let's think about what we are trying to do – do you think you might try it this way?' or some similar phrasing. Additionally, it is good for the self-esteem of the participants to highlight individual creativity and to share innovative ideas with the rest of the group.

Knowledge of Self
It is clear that you yourself – your personality, your attitude, your style of teaching, your experiences past and present, and how you are feeling at that particular time – will affect the session. There will be days when you know that the session did not go as well as it could have done. This could have been due to many varying factors, one of which might have been that your own feelings at the time were communicated unintentionally to the participants. This is not a sign of failure – it should be recognised and accepted as a transient expression of self. We say that, as part of our Sherborne skill base, we need to be able to observe individuals or the group and have the ability to read and respond to the 'messages' that come to us; it is just as likely that the people we are working with will be equally skilled at reading messages coming from us!

Knowledge of Helpers
Before starting a session, it is important to know what help will be required and where that help is coming from. When additional helpers are to be used, they should have the opportunity of taking part in movement sessions before they start to work with the participants, as this will help to give them an understanding of what is involved. This is particularly beneficial when participants become creative in their movement, and have ideas which can be developed, or where the group may be of very mixed abilities and needs, and 'individual work' is more beneficial. Given this knowledge and experience, the helper is in a position to respond individually to the needs of a participant who may be having problems with joining in specific group activities by engaging him in movement experiences that are more appropriate for him. If this should be the case, however, it is important to bring that person back into the group once the activity changes to one that is found to be acceptable to him.

Content and Timing of a Session
Content of a Session
Each session should contain experiences that focus on the following elements: body awareness, spatial awareness and relationships, the facility to experience varying movement qualities and the opportunity for creativity. It is important to note that some of the movements may well be the same for more than one of these elements. However, the language used to accompany the activity will focus on the concept being explored. For example, considering the movement 'sliding on stomachs': if it is being used as a body awareness activity, the accompanying dialogue might be: 'Can you feel your stomach [tummy/the front of your body] sliding over the floor? Can you make your body make wiggly lines as it slides over the floor?'; whereas, if the same movement were being used in a spatial context, the dialogue might be: 'Where are we? We are *low* down on the floor. Can you slide over the floor, keeping your body as low as possible? Can you find a spot across the room that is low down? Slide across to it keeping very low.'

An analysis of the vast majority of the movements in Sherborne's repertoire show that they can fit into more than one of the basic elements of her work; many also contain examples of more than one movement quality, which can add a depth to the experiences we offer. However, it is advisable to offer the experiences in straightforward, simple terms during sessions, as too much analysis will result in confusion. It is for us, as session leaders, to be aware of the underlying concepts of Sherborne's work in order to be in a position to offer an all-round, enriching experience to our group participants. Whenever possible, we need to allow the participants to be creative, developing their ideas in line with our own focused direction. Within the experiences, there should be a balance of individual and relationship work, opportunities for experiencing opposites of energy levels and movement qualities, together with periods of quiet and relaxation.

There are times when our movement session will have an open format, where the sequence of activities will be allowed to evolve freely and flexibly. At other times, the session can have a 'theme' within which the experiences are 'guided', whilst still allowing for flexibility and creativity. Such 'themes' might be 'strong and light movements' or 'sliding – incorporating pushing and pulling'; 'pathways through space – moving in straight and curving lines' might be a spatial theme for another session. 'Fast and slow' movements offer ample opportunity to explore different ways of travelling. It is quite possible to see how movement sessions, which include something of each of the elements of Sherborne's work, can be organised to stay within a designated theme.

When planning a balanced movement session, the following considerations may prove helpful. We need to ask ourselves:

1. What part of the body is moving? (Body awareness)

2. Where is the body moving? (Spatial awareness)

3. In what interactive context is the person moving – alone, with another person or with a group of people? (Relationships)

4. How is the body moving? (Movement quality)

Laban's movement analysis can further help us in planning the content of our movement sessions (see Table 4.1 below).

At first, we may not be confident enough to let a session 'evolve' or develop freely. We may feel that we need a list to work to. 'What if I dry up? What if I can't think of what to do next? If I let the participants have some influence over what happens next, will the session get out of control?', are very real concerns at the beginning of our experience with leading movement sessions. Again, this is not a sign of failure or incompetence. We might well need 'the list' in the early stages – I used to write one on the back of my hand! – but, as we extend our experience, our confidence will grow, and we will eventually be able to dispense with it. If the movement is new to all of us – session leaders and participants – we will 'grow' together as we share the activities, gaining confidence in our respective roles as the sessions progress.

Table 4.1 An Analysis of Movement
(based on the work of Rudolf Laban; printed with the permission of The Sherborne Association UK)

THE BODY What moves/What it does	**SPACE** Where the body moves
THE WHOLE BODY Stepping – Sliding – Turning – Vaulting – Rolling – Jumping – Gesture – Climbing – Crawling – Stillness INDIVIDUAL BODY PARTS Can lead Can support Can relate Can move symmetrically Can move asymmetrically	LEVELS High – Medium – Low DIRECTIONS Forward/Backward Diagonally/Sideways Up/Down Various Pathways: Curved – Straight – Zigzag RANGES Body Shapes: Wide/Narrow – Curved/Straight Body Spaces: Self/General Body Extensions: Near/Far – Large/Small
DYNAMICS/EFFORT/QUALITY How the body moves	**RELATIONSHIPS** Moving with objects/people
TIME Fast – Sustained – Slow – Sudden – Medium FORCE/WEIGHT Strong/Firm Fine touch/Light SPACE Direct/Straight Flexible/Circuitous FLOW Bound Free	OBJECTS Over/Under In/Out Between/Among In front/Behind Lead/Follow Above/Below Through/Around PEOPLE Mirroring Shadowing In Unison Together/Apart Alternating Simultaneously Partner/Group

Timing

As in all activities, timing is very important. The length of each session and the frequency of the sessions are important considerations. Ideally, a daily movement session is the best option; however, this may not be practical, but the minimum should be once a week. There is one particular aspect of SDM which cannot be emphasised too strongly. In terms of frequency of sessions, whatever the interval in between, sessions *must* be run on a regular basis, over a period of time, if the full benefits of the work are to be realised. To have the 'odd' movement session from time to time, or simply to run the sessions whenever they can be fitted in, will not result in positive outcomes in the fullest sense. If sessions are run on a regular basis, then, in the vast majority of cases, changes in responses and behaviour will become apparent.

As part of a video which I made in 1998 called *Never Say Never*, I have evidence of a group of approximately fifteen 6–9-year-old children with severe learning difficulties, who were abounding in energy, and therefore very active, whose 'movement' behaviour changed dramatically over a six-week period. Week one saw the children in a very 'free-flow' situation – running, jumping, twisting and, in some cases, self-excluding, working very much on an 'individual' basis. By the third week, they were beginning to come together in a 'loose circle' group, sharing body awareness and spatial activities, and, in some cases, giving each other slides. By week six, they had become a cohesive group, helping to make a tunnel for their friends to slither through, or helping to make a strong platform which friends could lie on to be swayed and rocked, and each patiently waiting their turn to 'have a go'; by this time, those who had self-excluded had become fully integrated members of the group. The sessions were led by four adults who, in the first instance, were prepared to 'meet the children where they were' – playing with them and allowing them a great deal of energetic freedom. This 'energy' was gradually structured so that eventually the sessions took on a much more constructive character and teachers were able to encourage co-operation and a sense of 'working together'.

The length of a session can vary from 15 minutes to an hour dependent on the ability and level of dependence of the participants. In some circumstances, five minutes may well be all that is needed; for example, for the first introductory session, or in response to the reaction of the participants. The length of each activity should be flexible to allow for the different speeds at which people work. Within the overall time constraints of the session, participants should be allowed to complete the movement experiences in their own time. This is an important consideration, which allows for the fact that we do not all work at the same speed. Some of us work quickly and therefore tend to 'finish' very quickly, whereas others take much longer. We need to respect these differences within our movement sessions. There is no harm in some of us waiting quietly whilst others complete their turn, as long as we know there will be something interesting happening after the wait. It also helps us to appreciate the differing characteristics we have as individuals, and gives us the opportunity to practise respecting differences in others.

During 'against' relationship activities, 'timing' can be quite critical. We need to be aware of what is happening and, if necessary, stop the activities before frustration and/or anger become apparent. There are many of us who need to experience what it is like to be strong and assertive without aggression, but, for some, if these experiences are allowed to continue too long without amicable resolve, the situation can become too demanding and 'determination and concentration' can become frustration. It is important that we monitor 'against' relationships and organise such activities carefully. For the majority of us, they are great fun, and should be treated as such. That some of us may have problems with them is no reason for not doing them; on the contrary, it is those very people who need to practise being strong in a positive, but non-aggressive way – possibly with ourselves or another 'helper' as a partner in the first instance.

In general terms, the timing of movement experiences will depend very much on the observation of responses that come from the group. At first, you may have to decide for yourself when to stop and change an activity, but, again, with experience, you will learn to 'read' the group or the individual you are working with, and their response will tell you when it is the time to change. For some of us, this 'growing awareness' of the group dynamics will come very quickly, almost at once; for others it may take longer. Again this is not a sign of failure or incompetence – give yourself and the individuals or group you are working with 'time to grow together'.

Starting and Finishing a Session
Starting a Session
Having decided through assessment who is going to take part, it is important to prepare the participants for these sessions. Each of the participants should be introduced to their particular helper if that person is not already known to him, told what is planned, what they will all be doing, and where they will be doing the activities. For some participants, it may be their first encounter with working on the floor or mats; the first session could well be involved with just these introductions, simply getting used to the idea, and sharing very simple movements together.

When starting the session, avoid being directive by inviting the participants to join you and the group on the floor, rather than telling them to come. In the first instance, it is important that everyone should be encouraged to be comfortable and feel relaxed. The start of the session could well be significantly different for children and adults. In general terms, less inhibited children will be able, with exceptions, to cope with relationship play, whereas adults will be more likely to need to come to terms with sharing space, taking part in individual body awareness and spatial activities, during which they can work without making physical contact with other participants in the first instance.

To reiterate, it is very important to start 'where the participants are'. A child with attention deficit/hyperactivity disorder will not come and sit with a partner/helper on the floor immediately. He will need a degree of freedom and play to start with and to be 'grounded' gradually with swinging and sliding – fast energetic activities; a young adult may not wish to make physical contact with another person; a child or young person on the autistic spectrum will be very unlikely to allow himself to be contained at first, and, for some of these people, perhaps never. People who are 'touch sensitive' may be encouraged to join in if our contact with them is made through another medium such as blankets, hoops or ropes. It is essential that we accommodate the varying needs of the group participants and allow the potential participants to 'let us in' or let themselves become involved in the session.

Finishing a Session
The closing of a session is as important as its beginning. Even though we may have started with individual movement experiences, it is important to bring the group together to finish and to allow everyone to relax and quieten down. *Quietness and stillness are as important as their opposite qualities which use a lot of energy and can, legitimately, be quite noisy at times.* To end the session, with everyone sitting quietly in a group, it is sometimes appropriate to play quiet music or to sing. At this point, it is important to ensure that each participant is acknowledged and thanked for taking part in the session. The coming together as a group at the end is significant in that it heightens our awareness of being a member of a group, and the fact that we have been sharing time and space together. Finding an appropriate way of getting back to shoes and socks, and not allowing it to happen in an ad hoc fashion, is also part of the run down of the session before safely leaving the room or hall and moving on to the next activity or journey.

Safety
Safety of the Environment
Before we begin the movement session, it is important that the surface of the floor is carefully examined. There have been instances in my experience of broken glass, drawing pins and other potentially dangerous objects left on the floor, especially when the space is also used for other activities. When the floor being used is wooden, there is always the possibility of splinters. Quite often, the hall being used doubles as a dining room, and therefore spillages need to be taken care of, as well as general cleaning. These may often seem to be quite trivial matters, but can be of major importance to someone who is about to lie on and slide on the floor! Attention must also be given to other equipment which might be in the hall/room. Often, there are stacks of chairs, benches, climbing apparatus and mats, and other furniture which, if not stacked or stored correctly, can be very hazardous in a situation which intentionally allows for energetic and at times fast-moving activities. It is prudent to check the area to be used for movement *before* the participants arrive.

Safety of Participants and Helpers/Supporters
Before introducing participants with physical disabilities to SDM, check, wherever possible with the physiotherapist, what range of movements is safe for the individuals and those which should be avoided. Always make sure that movements are carried out safely, and that there are enough helpers for experiences which involve supporting and lifting.

All session leaders and supporting helpers should be aware of safe lifting techniques. 'Lifting' is a major issue, both for participants and supporters, and is one of the major considerations when working with people with severe physical difficulties who are unable to move for themselves. The use of hoists for getting folks in and out of wheelchairs, down on to the floor and back up again can help facilitate access to Sherborne's work, but it has to be acknowledged that these processes are *very* time consuming. If there are not sufficient resources in terms of time, able bodied and strong helpers, and equipment, then the majority of the time allocated to the session can be taken up with just these things. If this happens, the session could be seen as being of little benefit to the participants and frustrating for the supporters.

The issue of 'lifting' can be prohibitive in terms of access for older people with profound and multiple learning difficulties; with small children, it is not such a big problem, although helpers must still look after their own bodies as well as those of the participants. However, if it is at all possible to involve older participants in SDM, then the benefits are tremendous. From being in a virtually constant 'bound state' in a wheelchair, sometimes with additional restrictions in terms of appliances, to being allowed access to 'free-flow' movement such as swinging in a blanket, being given a slide on a blanket (pulled by two people if necessary), being supported by someone else and rocked gently from side to side, must be a very enjoyable experience.

At all times, even when working with more able groups, we need to be particularly vigilant and observant in terms of safety when facilitating relationship activities. 'Safety' is a major issue, and rightly so, in any area where we are responsible for the well-being of others. It is an issue which, in my opinion, has to be addressed realistically, weighing up the advantages, disadvantages and reasonable risk factors within any given activity, if we are to offer what we believe to be rich, enhancing and beneficial experiences to the people we are working with.

The Issue of Touch

The issue of 'touch' falls, for me, within this area of thought. It is a major issue of our time, and one that cannot be ignored. Where there is an intransigent, 'no touch' policy, then there is absolutely no scope for the use of Sherborne's ideas, and that has to be respected and acknowledged. However, there is room for discussion and debate around the subject, and, at this point, I will outline some 'findings' which support the need for 'touch' in terms of the developing personality and well-being of individuals.

In Sylva and Lunt's book, *Child Development: A first course*, there is reference to the work of Bell and Ainsworth and their investigations into crying in babies in which it is pointed out that:

> *... the single most important factor which reduced crying... was the promptness with which a mother responded (usually by picking up or*

cuddling). The mother's early responsiveness and sensitivity to her baby's needs appeared to lay the foundations for the child's later social and emotional development. (Sylva and Lunt, 1986, p. 45)

... mothers who gave relatively more physical contact (cuddling and picking up) to their children in the early months, had children who enjoyed interaction with adults and were also happy to be put down and to turn cheerfully to exploration or play. (Ibid., p. 46)

I accept that this particular investigation focused on work with young babies; however, the fundamental need for physical touch is, in my opinion, a continuing basic need inherent in all of us. In the document, *Using the SEN Code of Practice – For the early years*, which has been produced by South Gloucestershire County Council, on the subject of 'rewards', it is pointed out that 'attention is the biggest reward of all', and the reward that is suggested is 'a hug'.

The problem, I think, is that as we get older, in certain cultures, response to this fundamental need is gradually eased out of us. When we are in our infant years, it is usually quite acceptable to have a cuddle, to hug another person or to put an arm around the shoulder as a sign of friendship and/or affection. Sadly, as we begin to 'grow up', this can come to be seen as 'socially inappropriate' or 'childish'. We keep each other at arm's length just in case our actions are misinterpreted. I believe that, even as adults, physical contact between family and friends remains a fundamental need in all of us. However, I totally accept that as we grow into adulthood there is a need to learn the distinction between behaviours which are appropriate, and those which are not, within varying relationships.

Conveying to someone else the sense of their being valued, being secure, being wanted and accepted, offering comfort in times of unhappiness and distress, sharing joy, and, basically, emphasising their 'belonging' is greatly enhanced if words are accompanied by some kind of appropriate physical contact. As we begin to grow through infancy into adolescence and adulthood, we still need situations in which physical contact is there at appropriate times to give us these feelings of security, value, belonging and acceptance. This is especially so if, for any reason, we do have feelings of insecurity or vulnerability, or are in need of reassurance or, just as importantly, for the sheer joy and positiveness of it! SDM gives us the opportunity legitimately and appropriately to revisit those childhood experiences and to explore the notion of appropriate behaviour at appropriate times.

Having said that, however, two words in particular, in the previous paragraph, immediately bring to mind the issue of touch – those words are 'insecurity' and 'vulnerability'. It would be totally wrong to dispute that it is a major issue of our time, and one that cannot be ignored. That many establishments working with young and often very vulnerable people do so under a 'no touch' regime is quite understandable. However, I would argue that the importance of 'touch' is so fundamental to the human psyche that, where possible, every effort should be made to create controlled, safe environments where work involving physical contact can be undertaken. I do accept that this is a *very* contentious issue, and that the safety of the people we are working with is *paramount*. On the other hand, I would also argue that we have a professional duty which requires us to provide what we believe to be the most beneficial and enriching experiences, in terms of personal development in all aspects, for the people we are working with, and it is our responsibility to ensure that the environment is 'safe'.

I accept that SDM cannot happen in a 'non-touch' environment; there is no argument about that. I do accept that there is a need for vigilance in any situation where close physical contact with others is involved, especially where there is additional outside help, or where the movement experiences are first being introduced to either group participants or supporters. However, my personal view is that the arguments for its inclusion in terms of the many advantages and benefits endemic within SDM outweigh those for its exclusion. Given convincing and strong arguments, there are circumstances, even where hard and fast policies have been laid down, where prescribed touch can be negotiated.

SDM usually happens in a group situation, which, in itself, offers considerable protection. In some therapeutic situations where work is more likely to be carried out on an individual basis, there may be provisions within the relevant policy which would allow SDM to take place (e.g. for another adult to accompany the SDM leader or observe them with the child through a 'one-way mirror'). In circumstances where there is difficulty or lack of clarity, it may be advisable to make parents or responsible carers aware of the fundamental aspects and benefits of SDM before the sessions begin.

Safe Use of Equipment
Very little equipment is used in SDM, but any which is being used needs to be checked out before the session begins. As has been pointed out earlier, the floor space needs to be clean and checked for any bits and pieces which might be lying about on the surface, and blankets which might be used for swinging and sliding need to be strong and safe. Shoes, wherever possible, should be removed, not only because this is desirable in terms of awareness and sensory input through our feet, but also in terms of safety, where close physical contact and support work may accidentally result in someone being hurt if heavy shoes are being worn. If shoes are worn, they should be of a lightweight style and material. Keeping socks on can be dangerous in terms of slipping. Due to the nature of the activities, it is appropriate for everyone to wear some kind of sports clothing, trousers or joggers. This may sound like stating the obvious, but I have witnessed SDM sessions where the girls and young ladies are working in skirts and dresses.

Implementing SDM with Varying Groups
Meeting Varying Needs
So far in this chapter, we have considered some aspects which apply to SDM sessions in general. The assessment of participants' strengths and needs, the content of a movement session, and safety factors as they apply to group participants, supporters and equipment, are applicable to all sessions, regardless of who is taking part. However, when we discussed 'starting a session', we began to consider how this might vary according to the intrinsic nature of the individuals who make up the group, and how we might help to make SDM accessible for individuals with attention deficit/hyperactivity disorder or who are on the autistic spectrum. Given the way in which the experiences are introduced to such individuals, once they become familiar with the approach used during the session, it may be surprising in some instances how involved the participants become. Within the psyche of the hyperactive child, who at first gives the impression of wanting to move only in fast, sudden, 'free flow' movements, there may be a desperate need to be 'contained' and to feel physically safe and secure. Once such a person has become 'grounded' and will allow himself to be 'contained', the tempo of the activities can be slowed down and other movement activities can be introduced.

Although during my time in special education, pupils and students with severe difficulties and profound and multiple learning difficulties have been the main focus of my attention, both in the classroom and during my SDM sessions, within those class groups there were often one or two individuals who had varying degrees of autistic spectrum disorder (ASD). With these individuals, I have found that the approach has to be ultra sensitive. It is often necessary to wait for the individual to 'let you in' on their terms and to devise ways of introducing movement experiences which will perhaps avoid eye-contact and physical touch with the use of blankets, hoops and ropes if necessary.

Accepting that there are some individuals for whom SDM is not a suitable or acceptable experience, I would suggest that it is the level of support, in many cases, which is crucial to a successful outcome or otherwise to the session. Certainly, in the first instance, each participant will need to work on a 1:1 basis. Working in this way will allow the helper to respond individually to each participant. As the sessions progress, individual needs and preferences in terms of the movement experiences will be noted. There is no reason why there should not be several different activities going on concurrently, if this is felt to be appropriate at the time, providing everyone comes back into the group at intervals during the session. This highlights the need, outlined in the 'Knowledge of Helpers' section above, for helpers to have an awareness of SDM prior to taking part in sessions. With this awareness of the movement, they will be able to respond individually to the actions and indications which come from the people with whom they are working.

More recently, I have been given the opportunity to work much more closely and intensely with pupils and students who have profound ASD. I am presently involved in a three-year research project which is being run collaboratively between Sunfield School in the West Midlands, a residential school for children and young people with ASD, and The Sherborne Association UK. The research is focused on 'Developing Social Engagement through Movement' (See Chapter 9).

The need for 'structure' when working with pupils/students with ASD is contrary to the very flexible and open approach normally associated with SDM sessions. We have been working to set programmes made up of movement experiences from Sherborne's repertoire which, over a period of time, have gradually become familiar to the participants. It would not be prudent at this stage either to describe in great detail the research project or to discuss at length any predicted trends or results, as at the time of writing there is still a considerable period of time before completion. However, I can say that, from a personal point of view, the levels of engagement that we have been able to achieve have been well above my expectations. Pupils who have previously been deemed as almost completely tactile defensive will now allow themselves to take part in all of the movement experiences offered to them; others who have been reluctant to give eye-contact now do so, either spontaneously or on request, whilst others are beginning to instigate their own movement responses or even take the initiative to lead the activities. Of course, there are still those who have not as yet taken an active part in the sessions, but I think this will always be the case for some participants in some sessions.

It is interesting to note that the particular groups of pupils/students who were selected to take part in the project were made up of those who were considered to have the most challenging behaviour patterns. The results of this particular piece of research will, it is envisaged, make a very significant case for the use of SDM with pupils with ASD to facilitate social engagement, communication and curriculum access.

The physical needs of participants who have profound and multiple learning difficulties dictate a very different approach. In the main, they are not able to make gross motor movements for themselves, and so we need to ask ourselves, 'How, under the circumstances, can we involve them in the "experience" intrinsic within particular movements?' For example:

- 'How can I give my partner the spatial experience of travelling in straight and wavy lines?' *By sliding them on a blanket.*
- 'How can I give my partner the experience of being curled up and contained?' *By wrapping my body around them, and talking about being small and wrapped up.*
- 'How can we share the experience of "going under a bridge"?' *By me pulling my partner on a blanket under a bridge made by another friend.* (In this case, it is important that I also go *under* the bridge as part of the shared activity.)

When working with small people, Sherborne spoke of *our* bodies becoming a 'second floor', so that we take our young partners on journeys on our tummies or on our backs. With imagination, it is possible to see that people with severe physical difficulties can be given the opportunity to become involved in many of Sherborne's experiences. Again, the level of available support is critical if these sessions are to be meaningful, beneficial and *safe*. It must be acknowledged, however, that there are even more constraints in terms of safety and support, as we have already discussed, if the people we are working with are physically big and heavy.

Although each session needs to be planned according to the strengths and needs of the individuals who make up that group, there are some key factors and general guidelines, in terms of organisation and support, which can help us in our planning, but, as with all aspects of SDM, there are no absolute rules (see Table 4.2 below).

We have so far been considering SDM as applicable to people with special needs and disabilities; however, a further, less obvious use of Sherborne's ideas is as a 'team-building' activity. George Hill writes that:

> *Based on my experience in higher education…[See Chapter 6] I was able to offer SDM as an option for team-building days. Several teams made up of social workers, staff from residential units and day centres took up this opportunity very successfully. Through the building up of positive relationships and trust in a non-challenging way, SDM offers a very satisfying team-building experience, by helping people to appreciate and enhance their own positive abilities whilst at the same time being able to see and acknowledge the positive aspects of their fellows.*

In this case, all of the participants were adults who were physically capable of looking after themselves. Although the sessions began with individual work, once confidence in the group situation had become established, the activities focused on 'relationship' experiences. All the aspects and principles of an SDM session, already discussed, were applied in exactly the same way as for the groups with young people with special needs. This use of SDM illustrates yet another way in which Sherborne's approach can be used. In general terms, the movement experiences remain the same; it is the modes of delivery, implementation, the language used and the focus of the session which vary according to the needs of the participating group members.

Table 4.2 (below) summarises how the implementation and organisation of movement sessions can be varied in order to meet the needs of differing groups. (The numbers and ages are for guidance only.)

Table 4.2 Organisation of SDM sessions according to group need

GROUP CHARACTERISTICS	KEY FACTORS
Children with severe learning difficulties, approx. 6 years and upwards Mobile, able to move independently Able to work in a group with adult support	**Level of support:** Child:adult ratio, 3:1 **Focus:** All aspects of SDM. **Organisation:** Children working together where possible.
Children with severe learning difficulties, up to 6 years Having a degree of mobility	**Level of support:** Supported by 6–8 adults, working in a ratio of 1:1 **Focus:** All aspects of SDM, but mainly on relationships work. Mainly floor-based activities. **Organisation:** Work in groups with other children with adult support.
Children on the autistic spectrum, those with emotional and/or behavioural problems and challenging behaviour, all ages *Do not force any movement experience – the more you try this the more the child is likely to resist and to become distressed. It is better to change the activity.*	**Level of support:** Child:adult ratio, 1:1 **Focus:** Relationship work with adult. Mainly floor-based activities. **Organisation:** Work in a small group of 4–6 participants. Follow 'routine'. Introduce new experiences very gently. Be prepared to allow varying activities within group – according to individual responses. Give 'routine' cues to activities. Be prepared to use supporting materials, e.g. blankets, ropes, hoops, etc., especially with children who are tactile defensive.
Children with profound and multiple learning difficulties, up to approx. 12 years	**Level of support:** Child:adult ratio, 1:1 **Focus:** Using all aspects of SDM, with adult acting as physical support for sliding, rolling, swinging, etc. Free flow activities are most beneficial, e.g. swinging, sliding, etc. (using blankets). **Organisation:** Work in group.
Young adults with profound and multiple learning difficulties, 12 years and upward	**Level of support:** As above, but with higher ratio of adult:participant support – 2:1. If there is a problem with the level of support needed, this may be overcome by working with one or two participants at a time, ensuring that the other participants are not kept waiting too long for their turn. Be aware of 'lifting' issues. **Focus** and **Organisation:** As above.
Children and young people with attention deficit/hyperactivity disorder	**Level of support:** Child:adult ratio, 1:1 **Focus:** High-energy active movements to start with (sliding, swinging, rolling, jumping, etc.). Keep activities focused on 'work with partner' – helpful to keep experiences floor-based as much as possible. **Organisation:** Work in small groups with 4–5 participants. Be prepared to change activity quickly. Gradually slow tempo of the session. End with 'quiet contained' experience. **Be prepared to give out a lot of energy!**

Teacher Qualities
Towards the end of her book, Sherborne lists what she considers to be some of the qualities necessary in a person who teaches SDM. Among those qualities, she includes emotional stability, the capacity to relate to the disturbed child, a sense of humour, the ability to play, and directness and honesty. These attributes allow us to relate positively to the participants with whom we are working in the emotionally and socially secure atmosphere discussed in Chapters 2 and 3.

In this chapter, we have been involved with the practical aspects of running SDM sessions. It is notable that Sherborne completes her list of 'qualities' with resilience and stamina! If we are to achieve positive outcomes to our movement sessions, it is *highly likely* that we are going to need plenty of both! We need the resilience to 'continue' beyond a beginning where we might not *appear* to be making a lot of progress. As already pointed out, the beneficial effects of SDM do not appear overnight or during the early sessions. Both we and group participants need time to internalise what is happening and then to respond; participants who may not appear to like some of the experiences often come to enjoy them if they continue to be presented in a non-threatening, sensitive way. Professionally, we may need to have the resilience to continue with the work amid scepticism from colleagues who may not understand the principles of the work. To look into a hall where children are 'rolling on the floor', trying with all their might to push *you* over may not look too professional to the uninitiated! You have to be very brave and resolute to keep going – but keep going you will if you have the resilience and absolute belief in what you are doing. Maybe you will inspire colleagues to become interested enough to want to know more about the work, and even become involved. 'Stamina', we certainly need. Running an SDM session with a group of lively children, brimming with energy, takes a great deal of our own energy especially if the participants are at the stage where they still need 1:1 support. Supporting sessions for children or older people with multiple needs also takes a tremendous amount of stamina.

This all sounds very 'energetic'. Is there a need to be 'super fit' to run SDM sessions? No, there is not! Providing we are reasonably well and fit, our enthusiasm and motivation makes us *want* to offer the people we are working with an enriching and beneficial on-going experience that is both enjoyable and fun. This will provide us with the energy, resilience and stamina necessary to undertake the work.

References
Sherborne, V. (2001) *Developmental Movement for Children: Mainstream, special needs and pre-school* (2nd edn). London: Worth Publishing.
South Gloucestershire Council (2002) *Using the SEN Code of Practice for the Early Years – Guiding Principles: Part 4 – Managing behaviour*. Local publication: South Gloucestershire Council.
Sylva, K. and Lunt, I. (1986) *Child Development: A first course*. Oxford: Blackwell.

CHAPTER 5
Sherborne Developmental Movement in the Community and in Therapy

Introduction

The range of applications of Sherborne Developmental Movement (SDM) described in this chapter by a number of international practitioners illustrates the 'broadening perspective' referred to in the subtitle of this book. As I have already described, Sherborne developed her ideas mostly in the field of Special Education, but latterly her work has taken on a great deal of importance in many other settings, including work in the community and in therapy. As my experience has also been mostly in special education, I felt I needed to call on the expertise of people working in these other environments, whose work with SDM I have known and respected for many years.

I have included a brief introduction to each of the writers – Janice Filer, Penny Rance, the multidisciplinary team of Belgian therapists and Chris Handley – at the beginning of this book.

SDM and its Role in Family Therapy
Dr Janice Filer

Developmental Movement Play is an innovative early intervention programme that addresses the needs of two generations by providing a service for the child and parent. It is a group work practice that uses movement, incorporating SDM as part of a programme to address issues concerning communication, relationships, and emotional, behavioural and mental health difficulties for parents and children during the early years.

Developmental Movement Play evolved from my practice as a teacher of Physical Education (PE) and my work in a nursery school. There I used SDM as the basis for dance and movement workshops which were set up to encourage positive parent/school partnerships. Many of these groups involved parents of toddlers and young children who were having trouble with language, social skills, making relationships, and setting and keeping boundaries. Parents were experiencing difficulties bonding and making relationships with their children, playing with them and using any form of positive behaviour management.

The origins of dance and movement as a healing art lie in ancient history. Dance and movement are the most fundamental of all the arts, as they involve the direct expression of oneself through the body – which is a basic form of communication. They allow a natural way of working with very young children, as every child has its own natural inner rhythm and can move in some way.

Developmental Movement Play is the psychotherapeutic use of movement and dance through which a person can engage creatively in a process to further their emotional, cognitive, physical and social integration. It is based on the principle that movement reflects an individual's patterns of thinking and feeling. There are no steps to learn, and participants learn to listen to themselves through moving. The dance is different every time, as they are constantly changing and moving in unique ways, expressing themselves in a movement language that comes from the core of their being. Developmental Movement Play appears to be a simple practice, yet its effects are powerful and profound. It gives parents and children permission to feel what they are feeling. By accepting their feelings, participants are able to work through them within the safe boundaries of the movement activities.

In keeping with Sherborne's work, there are three key elements to Developmental Movement Play that make it effective as a therapeutic intervention. These are the importance of holistic vision, an affective climate and the basic style of interaction of the movement teacher. Throughout, the child is considered in the context of the whole person. Attention is focused on their self-confidence, self-esteem, and sense of competence, well-being and pleasure in their own ability – the personality concepts that are part of the whole child. These concepts form the basis for learning and growing in any area of development. They are not divided up into separate disciplines, but dealt with as a whole.

Developing Positive Relationships

In Developmental Movement Play, the starting point is the development of relationships through movement for both parent and child – in particular the relationship with 'self', and their relationship with each other. The focus is on providing them with practical dance and movement experiences which enable them to repair and enhance their attachment relationship, alongside improving self-esteem and body image, and developing effective communication skills as the basis from which to enter into relationships with others.

Parents are inherently defensive about their child's behaviour because they are so closely identified with each other; therefore, the intervention is focused on the play relationship between parent and child rather than on difficult behaviours. Through Developmental Movement Play, parents are encouraged to put positive parenting skills into practice with their child, at the time of learning, in a safe, controlled environment with the encouragement and support of trained helpers. Parents and children learn all about realistic expectation, boundary-setting, and using positive language and commands, whilst having fun and enjoying each other through shared movement activities. They learn together as they play together. Thus, relationship play assists in developing closeness and communication between parent and child.

The Importance of Touch

Developmental Movement Play is a simple way to establish a deeper emotional parent–child bond. During sessions, emphasis is on developing a trusting relationship through activities which give them the opportunity to practice safe, sensitive, physical contact. Parents are given the opportunity to express love through loving-caring-touching relationship play with their child. Leboyer in his book, *Loving Hands: The traditional art of baby massage* (1977), says:

> It is through loving, caressing, tactile stimulation and communication that the infant learns that he/she is loved... We must speak to their skins. We must speak to their backs, which thirst and cry as much as their bellies.

Studies show that babies who are held, massaged, carried and rocked grow into adults who are more compassionate and co-operative, and are less aggressive and violent.

Developmental Movement Play leads to pleasure and relaxation for both parent and child. Parents find it provides positive and cyclic reinforcement of their parenting abilities to love and care for their child, as well as increasing their confidence in handling and relating to them. Making loving touch a regular part of family life, and watching the effect it has on a child's sense of well-being, security and confidence, is a joy to see.

Listening to Children

Not all children are listened to in their relationship with their parents. There may be little or no conversation in a family. Children may be talked at, ignored and have little opportunity to express feelings in order to make themselves understood. Through Developmental Movement Play, parents learn how to notice and to listen to their child's non-verbal cues. When a child is listened to wholeheartedly, relationships – both with self and other – begin to change for the better.

Some children and parents find it too difficult to connect through eye-contact due to the difficulties they have already experienced in their relationship. Gentle touch can be used to overcome this problem. The trained movement teacher will encourage parents to pick up on non-verbal cues and to experiment with less threatening ways of communication until they and their child have built up the level of mutual trust necessary to give each other eye-contact or to face each other. Many of the Developmental Movement Play activities can be adapted to work in a side-by-side or back-to-back position until this trust builds up.

The Role of the Parent

The structure of the Developmental Movement Play group helps to create the climate that provides the child and parent with a safe, secure environment, where positive encouragement enables independent exploration and learning to take place. The parent is guided through the movement activities by the teacher, who enables them to build on their own positive experiences in order to provide them for their child. Well planned dance and movement experiences that focus on touch enable the parent to experience and understand fully the importance of the gentle but firm touch which deepens the feeling between parent and child, and the sensitivity of handling that a young child needs to feel safe enough for attachment to take place. During Developmental Movement Play, there is scope to encourage and practise the gentleness of touch that some parents need to experience themselves before they are able to handle their child appropriately. It brings about a breakthrough in that negative cycle of experiences for both parent and child, leading to a relationship that enables the parent to feel more loving towards the child and the child more lovable.

The parent is encouraged to share, with the teacher and other participants, the responsibility of creating an environment in which the children experience respect, acceptance and enjoyment of their own possibilities. In developing this shared sense of practice, the movement teacher guides and supports the parents in achieving this aim within the supportive structures of the group.

Developmental Movement Play provides opportunities for parents to grow as individuals alongside their offspring. The weekly rehearsing of adaptive coping behaviours enables the parent to continue activities at home so they can bring about small positive changes in the nurturing of their children.

The Movement Teacher

As with any therapeutic work, it is essential that the movement teacher is emotionally secure and is able to adopt a non-critical approach when working with the participants. Movement sessions must be filled with warmth, affection and fun so that the activities provide learning experiences for children and their parents in a non-threatening atmosphere. It is crucial that the teacher is sensitive and responsive to the possibilities and the non-verbal interaction of both the child and parent.

It is also important that the movement teacher has previously taken part in practical dance and movement activities. To use Developmental Movement Play as a therapeutic intervention, we need to learn to be sensitive to the flow of energy within our bodies. We need to learn how to organise that energy, to focus, to direct it, to listen to our hearts and honour our need to express our feelings before we can provide the environment to encourage others to do the same. It is the first-hand, practical experience which leads to a deeper understanding of this work, and enables the teacher to use movement as a spiritual healing process which helps young children to become truly at home in their bodies.

Developmental Movement Play aims to give participants the opportunity to communicate in a non-verbal way through movement activities. All activities are developed from the leader's observation of individual need during each session. Observation and anticipation are key elements to the success of Developmental Movement Play. These elements enable the experienced movement teacher to create a climate in which a child experiences safety, appreciation and success, and in which children and their parents can begin to grow together. They must be able to anticipate the initiatives of the child, the child's reactions and the child's emotional expressions. This can take place only if the movement teacher has the experience and observational skills to assess what is happening with each individual in the group.

The Developmental Movement Play Session
The only way to understand this style of practice fully is to do it. Developmental Movement Play is very personal form of dance and movement that is not easily explained by words. All children and their parents can be included in the practice of Developmental Movement Play, regardless of their stage of development, physical ability, class or culture. Emotions and perceptions of disability are invited into the dance activities to be expressed and released as a natural part of what is happening in the sessions.

Participants are encouraged to take their time, and not to rush into anything until they feel comfortable. They are encouraged to go with what works for them. Sometimes sessions are easy and comfortable for people; sometimes they are challenging. Everything is dependent on the mood. Participants are encouraged to stay open to how they feel. They are also encouraged to be responsible for the well-being of their own body, and their own child or children.

The activities enable participants to become aware of themselves through a physical awareness of their body. Initially, development of physical awareness takes place through movement activities near the ground. In the beginning, there is an overriding need for participants to feel a sense of security. This is created by the containing ethos of the group and through the experience of more grounded movement, as most people feel safer working near to the floor.

Through better physical awareness, participants gradually gain better control of movement, better control of balance and better control of energy. These aspects of personal growth lead to greater self-confidence for both parent and child. Being at home in our bodies and honest in our emotions are aspects of our personalities which make us likeable and appealing to other people. This in turn leads to better interpersonal relationships. With this increasing development of sense of self, children begin to experience self-respect and self-worth. It is only then that children are able to begin to develop an awareness of others. This occurs first with the people the child is closest to, usually the mother. As children become increasingly aware of other people's needs, they begin to develop the ability to enter into relationships with them.

In Developmental Movement Play, children and their parents are encouraged to work individually, in pairs and in small groups. They are invited to move body parts such as head, shoulders or knees, focusing on the emotional energies contained in each part. They are gently steered towards becoming aware of what emotions they have stored and where they have stored them. They are encouraged to move their body according to how it feels on the day so that the body tells their story through movement. They are encouraged to become aware of their inner anger, which might present itself as tension in muscles or posture. As they become aware of their feelings, they develop the trust to allow their body to tell its own story through dance. In doing so, they release some of their inner tensions. They are encouraged to follow their feet and keep them moving until a force bigger than themself is causing the moving. If they are aware of any specific feeling, they are encouraged to express it by allowing it to move through their dance.

Over time, parents and children also develop the ability to listen to the movement of their inner body rhythms when silent and still. Once the anger has been released, a spiritual awareness develops when participants can seek solace and refuge as they connect to the deepest part of themselves. When they reach this point, they are ready to tackle one of the most difficult aspects of movement play – stillness. During stillness, participants have a tendency to hold their breath. The leader needs to be aware of this tendency and to keep track of it. When someone in the group is holding their breath, they need to be encouraged to let go. To counteract the tendency to hold breath, participants are encouraged to move until they cannot hold their breath any more and, by way of contrast, to repeat the movement activity while breathing to feel the difference. They are encouraged to stop moving to feel the dance; and to move in slow motion. They are called to rest after movement, and to close their eyes whilst they focus on the ebb and flow of their breathing, the beat of their heart, the inner pulsing of their body, as they embrace the stillness. Participants are encouraged to move as little as possible as they feel and listen to the rhythm of each other's bodies. This brings about a spiritual closeness for the parent and child.

The Developmental Movement Play Workshop

Requirements

- As no special equipment is necessary, any setting with a large enough space can be suitable as long as it is warm, light, airy and free from hazards. It is also useful if there is space for refreshments, as the social side of the group is important, and gives participants an opportunity to discuss any issues in an informal way.

- It is important that the venue itself is unthreatening. The most appropriate setting will differ depending upon the make-up of the group at the time. Nurturing participants – both children and parents – by providing an environment where they feel comfortable is as important as the Developmental Movement Play itself. The room should not be overlooked, as it is difficult for participants to let go of inhibitions when there are constant interruptions or an unwelcome audience.

- You may need some old, but strong, blankets for some activities.

Aim of the Workshop

- The aim is that parents come to the group to feel relaxed, and leave with a new skill to practise with their children at home.

Format of the Workshop Sessions

- The engagement process begins with a home assessment visit. Friendly, follow-up phone calls, home visits or letters, before and during the period of the workshops, keep participants on board.

- The Developmental Movement Play workshop runs for approximately 10 weeks; each full-length session lasts about two hours.

- The first, introductory session gives participants an overview of what to expect from the workshops, and a 'taste' of the Developmental Movement Play which lasts for about ten minutes. Parents and their children are then invited to join the group for two more taster sessions to find out more about it before they make a commitment to the full programme.

- The actual Developmental Movement Play period in each session lasts between 20 minutes and an hour depending on the need and mood of the group.

- The workshop begins with a sharing time, when parents have an opportunity to talk about their experiences as parents whilst their children enjoy soft play or other appropriate activities supported by the staff team.

- When the majority of children are ready to begin the session, the leader takes up a place in the circle of parents as a signal that the relationship play is about to start.

- The structured part of the workshop starts with the ritual singing or humming of a well-loved nursery rhyme or song to accompany the rocking activities, which are always included in the session. This rocking, cuddling time is always repeated as a calming activity at the end. Children and their parents learn and choose action songs as a base from which the 'Developmental Movement' takes place. Individual, partner and group activities develop according to individual or group need. This will include relationship play and blanket play. After calming down, children, parents and staff enjoy refreshments together before evaluating the day's programme.

- During refreshments, there is time for discussion about a relevant topic, such as weaning, sleeping, crying, returning to work, etc.

- The leader plans the work for each follow-up session from their observations of the previous session. Movement activities selected for this session should relate to children's movement schemas, their interests, moods and level of development and interaction with their parent.

Outcomes for Children
It is my experience that there are powerful outcomes for children from taking part in Developmental Movement Play, particularly in the areas of self-esteem, balanced relationships and developmental learning.

Improved Self-Esteem
By the ages of two or three years, some children have already developed a negative sense of self through life experience and inadequate parenting. The movement teacher acts as facilitator to the healing process through modelling and sensitive intervention. Providing an environment rich in positive experiences will enable both the child and parent to establish the sense of self-worth necessary for the development of relationship-building.

Developmental Movement Play addresses the issues of the negative downward spiral that occurs when a child sees himself as unlovable in relation to a hostile world of unloving people. Through the positive relationship experiences encouraged during Developmental Movement Play, the child's learned judgement – that he is good for nothing – will slowly begin to change, until he realises that there are times when he can be successful. As the child begins to feel more positive about himself, he begins to realise that he can be accepted for himself, that there are people who are kind and warm to others, and that the world might not be such a bad place after all.

Balanced Relationships
Developmental Movement Play works on two levels. Parents and children can explore and participate freely on an individual level within the context of the movement activity at the same time as working together. From observation of need, the teacher creates movement activities based on everyday movements such as rocking, cradling, supporting, containing, bouncing, rolling, swinging and sliding, as described in *Developmental Movement for Children* (Sherborne, 2001). These playful, everyday movement activities encourage a child to work with or alongside a parent who will give them security. Given this security, young children will naturally move to greater and more appropriate independence when they are developmentally ready. The time of readiness is determined by the child's level of self-confidence and emotional well-being. It does not occur at any specific age, particularly for children being raised in a traumatic situation.

In Developmental Movement Play, activities give both parent and child the opportunity to experience the struggle of their balance of power by shifting between taking the lead and being led, by trying out 'with' 'shared' and 'against' relationships. They both begin to accept that struggle is not altogether a bad thing but an innate part of the learning process. The child begins to understand that there are times when they can be in control of their life, as well as times when they are controlled by others; the parent learns how to handle the struggle and the gradual relinquishment of parental control through trying things out in the safe context of the group.

Developmental Learning
Developmental Movement Play helps children to manage feelings that interrupt learning. In Developmental Movement Play workshops, the focus is on the early relationship movement play between parent and child. The aim is to develop some of those early skills, termed 'the prerequisites to learning', when children are beginning to:

- Look and pay attention
- Communicate
- Relate
- Play
- Co-ordinate the body
- Overcome behavioural and emotional barriers.

Current research has shown that movement is the key to learning at any age. Our brains develop through everyday movements such as crawling, walking, running, climbing, turning, skipping and so on. Developmental Movement Play is based upon these everyday movements. The basic structure is therefore unthreatening to participants, as it is rooted in their usual movement patterns. In Developmental Movement Play, both sides of the brain are developed through structured movement activities which enable participants to create movement patterns in their own inimitable individual way. Throughout the Developmental Movement Play activities, children begin to learn to use the body as a creative and expressive instrument.

Outcomes for Parents
Significant outcomes for parents are often realised in the areas of the emotions, their mental health and their relationship with their child.

Emotional Liberation
Through movement, the body becomes a tool for creativity and energetic expression. Participants become receptive to an experience that can be touching, powerful, liberating, joyful and healing. It is this experience which enables the movement teacher to provide the scaffolding for them as they build on their own experiences. At a deeper, intuitive level, participants are able to let go and release inner emotions that sometimes remain unexpressed in daily life.

Improved Mental Health
In my experience, there are a number of mental health issues which are addressed by Developmental Movement Play, and my observations and video records demonstrate that participants experience improvement over time. For example, it is my experience that mothers with post-natal depression, who attend Developmental Movement Play classes, experience tangible benefits after only a few sessions. Post-natal depression not only harms the sufferer, but also can severely affect the bonding process between parent and child. It can also harm the future development of the infant, leading to mental health and behavioural problems. Improvements in the mother's health improve the child's life chances. Statistics show that one in seven pre-school children experience some kind of

mental health problem, and evidence highlighted by the Mental Health Foundation's *Bright Futures* report (1999) shows that early intervention programmes can be very effective in preventing this.

Both movement and dance are also powerful tools for stress management. The physical activity involved helps decrease the production of hormones associated with stress.

Improved Parent–Child Relationships
Some parents have expressed that, during the movement sessions, they experienced quality play with their child for the very first time, and that this was, in itself, a highly emotional experience for them. It is uplifting to witness this procedure as it takes place. To hear a mother saying through tears of joy during movement activities with her four-year-old son, 'This is the first time I have ever really played with my child, and I didn't realise what I was missing until now,' illustrates the level of success of the Developmental Movement Play approach.

Conclusion
To be able to feel at one with yourself in a shared experience with your child is joyous. The power of Developmental Movement Play is that it brings about change for both the parent and child together, enabling the child to be on the receiving end of positive experiences from the person who counts most during their early years – the parent. Using Development Movement Play as an early intervention which supports the strengthening of relationships between parents and children has enabled many families to overcome destructive patterns of past behaviour and negative relationships, and replace them with the positive relationship experiences learned during movement sessions. In the words of a parent who attended one of the first workshops, 'It's a great experience for parents and children together – lots of fun and excitement, boosts confidence… I cannot believe the change in [my child] or me.'

Although there has been no formal research carried out on the benefits of Developmental Movement Play for participants, I have amassed over the years a wealth of video evidence – I tape *all* my Developmental Movement Play sessions! These sequential recordings show exciting, positive developments for parents and children during the course of the workshop in many areas where they had specific issues. As a result of work with relationships, communication, emotional difficulties, self-image, mental health, loss, transition or change, lives have been altered and enriched.

Developmental Movement Play can also be used with participants of all ages, in a variety of settings and for a variety of reasons, not only as an early intervention to build parent–child relationships. It can be a way in which to touch the spiritual essence within others and ourselves. From the beginning of time, movement, story and song have brought people together.

References

Leboyer, F. (1977) *Loving Hands: The traditional art of baby massage.* London: Collins.

Sherborne, V. (2001) *Developmental Movement for Children: Mainstream, special needs and pre-school* (2nd edn). London: Worth Publishing.

Mental Health Foundation (1999) *Bright Futures: Promoting children and young people's mental health.* London: Mental Health Foundation.

SDM and Dance in the Community
Penny Rance

I discovered SDM in my specialist training in disability dance during the early 1990s. It appeared to me to be useful, relevant and appropriate, especially when measured against my own experiences as a mother of three children. I find that SDM approaches to understanding our bodies, through relationships and the force of gravity, underpin the majority of my dance work. This work takes place with people who have a range of disabilities, from those who are profoundly disabled through to those whose disability is invisible (e.g. hearing impairment, dyspraxia, autistic spectrum disorder (ASD)). Different groups reflect this variety – some integrated, some discreet, some across a small range of disability and some across a much wider range.

SDM is usually fitted into my dance sessions about a one-third of the way to halfway through. This is after the initial warm up, which is individual, and before the creative work or the more formal learning of a particular series of moves. I find SDM provides a useful structure for my sessions. It is not the only tool that I use, but it is what I come back to when the going gets tough. People have a choice as to whether they attend the sessions that I lead, so, to be assured of earning a living as well as having fun and enjoyment doing so, it is important that those who come to the sessions want to return (Csikszentimihalyi, 1992)! Thus they need to share the enjoyment and fun, but, to ensure the durability of this fun, there needs to be a structure. SDM helps me to provide this structure.

Below are three different examples of how I use SDM. The first takes place during a local, summer play-scheme for children with a very wide range of disabilities. The second is TAMBA, which is an integrated creative dance group. This group has been running now for over seven years, and three of the original members are still with us. The third example is from a school for children with moderate learning difficulties where I worked for a period of six weeks.

Summer Play-Scheme – 'Caring' Relationships
This is an annual provision – five days a week for four weeks during the summer holidays for local children with disabilities. The provision is taken up by over 30 children on any one day, and there is a high ratio of staff support. I go in about twice a week to work with some of the children during either the morning or afternoon session.

The group is open and self-selected, which means that anyone can drop in or out at any time. I tend to organise my sessions here to a basic pattern, so that children and support workers can work out what might be happening at any one scheduled point in the sessions. We have found, over the years, that the children with the highest level of disabilities appear to enjoy these sessions the most.

The most popular activity with the children, particularly for those in wheelchairs, is 'double rolling'. 'Double rolling' is a 'caring' relationship activity, thus I supply the energy. I lie on my back on a mat, with the child lying on top, so we are tummy-to-tummy. Where possible, their faces rest just over my shoulder with as much eye-contact as possible whilst getting into place. They have to hang on as tight as possible. Very carefully and slowly, I roll over, taking the child with me, actively sensing how they feel and watching their faces when possible. Obviously, I take my own weight when on top, but with just enough 'squash' factor to make it fun for the child. The organisation of arms and legs can be quite complex especially when working with a child with cerebral palsy, which describes most of the children who elect to join in this experience.

Every person who is not too big who wants a go gets one – two if I am feeling strong! If the children are too large, I stick to basic rolling; safety is important for everyone. We usually roll to the other side of the mats or to the other side of the circle, if there is one.

So what are the benefits? Well, most importantly it is fun, especially for children who are often very carefully cared for, because there is a tiny element of very well-controlled danger and consequent excitement. It is about being very closely involved with someone else, and experiencing gravity in a different way – defeating gravity on the upward part of the roll; being responsible for 'hanging on', and thus having a valid part to play in the experience; and 'falling' the smallest possible distance. Consequently, the children experience two types of movement – both free-flow and bound – in one activity, giving a greater range of movement sensations. This activity helps develop the physical sense of self through partnership with another, and an awareness of torso and hips, which is often difficult for children with disabilities to discover. Sometimes, this is the easiest way to introduce children to the sensation of rolling. They have physical reassurance along the length of their bodies from the care-giver, which helps them to relax, closely monitored by the care-giver. There is also the social aspect of turn-taking that is gained whilst being part of a larger group.

TAMBA – 'Sharing' and 'Against' Relationships
TAMBA is dance group for children with special needs and their siblings, aged 10 to 18 years. There are currently eight members and two leaders. The group is very able, and is supported by two student volunteers whose primary brief is to set a positive role model. The young people have been performing in local community events and on dance platforms for the past four years, and have developed a reputation for having a very special quality of movement and relationship within the group, rarely seen elsewhere. Needless to say SDM features heavily in our programme.

I shall describe the activities which supported the group's most recent work with 'shared' relationships, which then developed into work with 'against' relationships. The purpose of these two movement experiences was to prepare the group to work on a performance piece which explored relationships and opposition.

'Back-to-back rocking' is a 'shared' activity; the energy contributions from the partners are equal. The activity is gentle, and, once the individual rhythms are established, it is mutually enjoyable. I do not use music, and so the partners find their own pace – one that is right for both bodies. The benefits are an increased awareness of self through interaction with others, both physically and personally. It develops an understanding of the torso, and its function in supporting the body, and an increased sense of personal centre. The visibility of the limbs to the participants, and how they are utilised in this experience, aids the development of the sense of wholeness of their bodies.

Once the group was comfortable with this activity, I moved the movement experience onto an 'against' relationship to develop and strengthen the sense of centre further.

The 'against' activity we used is called 'rocks'. One person 'roots' themselves firmly to the floor – knees bent, legs spread to a comfortable angle, the soles of the feet flat on the floor; arms are placed slightly behind the line of the shoulders, with the hands spread on the floor. The object of the activity is for the 'rock's' partner to push them over.

For this particular movement experience, the adult care-givers worked with the more vulnerable members of the group. Like most sensitive care-givers, we all fell over, with much laughter, when sufficient effort had been made by our partners. By doing so, we ensured that they did not become disheartened. We also did not actually push our 'rocks' over, but, by pushing them gently, enabled them to sense their own centre more clearly and thus develop more strength. The remainder of the group were fairly evenly matched. There was much laughter when the rocks fell over, a lot of exhausted bodies lying on the floor and a great sense of relaxation and release. We also achieved my personal objectives: to confirm and enhance the relationships within the group and to strengthen individuals' sense of centre and awareness of their limbs.

There were three interesting outcomes. Everyone grasped and could perform this movement immediately, despite the fact that this was the first time that the group had experienced 'rocks'. A young lady with a brain tumour and partial paralysis down her left side was the best rock; she was immovable. She was also very good at moving other rocks, much to her apparent joy. Finally – and I still smile when I recall this event – one young lady with Down's syndrome had the wit to pick up my legs and roll me over, chuckling as she did so.

The School Setting – 'Against/Sharing' and 'Against' Relationships
This was a series of six regular workshops with two comparable classes of 9–10-year-old children with moderate learning difficulties. Some of the children had a boundless energy, which was manifesting itself in anti-social playground behaviours. For obvious reasons, I used the 'against' approach for part of these sessions to tap into this energy, and thus give the children a positive rather than negative experience of their own physicality.

There were about 12 children in each group, and I was supported by two staff, sometimes three. The initial plan for both classes was the same. As usual, the two groups evolved their own personalities very quickly, and unsurprisingly the higher energy group accessed the 'against' opportunities more fully.

The first movement experience I selected for the groups to work on was a 'Hand-to-hand push'. For this activity, the participants face each other, feet planted firmly on the floor, comfortably far apart, with strong bouncy knees leaning slightly towards their partners. They then push palm-to-palm with slightly extended arms. The idea is to match the partner's energy and to find a very strong position, a point of inertia, where neither is pushed over. The second part of the movement is to release from this position, taking care of self and partner, without falling over.

However, being aware that touch had not necessarily been used constructively in other circumstances, I first prepared the groups for this work using 'pass the touch'. I use this activity in many environments. It can be great fun, and I find it an excellent 'group building' tool.

I organised the group in a circle, and the task was to pass the 'touch' around it. Thus, there was the opportunity to do the movement and to watch others doing it (Smith-Autard, 1994). The object of the activity was for participants to pass whatever form of touch they received onto the person next to them, so that the touch went round the circle – a visual 'Chinese whispers'. I clearly indicated the direction the 'touch' would be travelling around the circle before we started the activity. To start, I gently touched the person next to me, using my index finger to their index finger, and they passed it onto the next person. The requirement of a gentle quality was stressed throughout this stage of the activity. The initial objective was to engender respect of individuals within the group for each other, and awareness of the whole group through the interaction with the people either side and watching people opposite perform a similar interaction. (Some people needed a gentle prompt to watch what was happening.) I also wanted them to build up a body knowledge of how their two neighbours functioned physically.

Generally, for this activity, the matching of the use of a particular body part is a requirement of the movement. This gives me a good idea of a person's awareness of their own body, and of their awareness that another person has a matching body part, and in some cases that there is another person. It also tells me whether people like and can accept touch, or are completely unhappy with it. In the latter case, I quickly substitute props, such as inflatable globes, beanbags, soft frogs, etc. I can also use this activity to 'warm up' a particular body part and awareness of it for a later movement; for example, backs wriggling against each other.

During the first week, I just progressed this activity to touching palm to palm. However, it was in the second week with the more energetic group, and in the third with the other, that I felt able to introduce the 'against' work. I decided which of my neighbours was the more able for this particular movement experience, and demonstrated to the group how we could push against each other palm-to-palm. We concentrated on keeping eye-contact and placing the feet well apart, one in front of the other, with strong, bent knees. There was an emphasis on a matching of strength. What was crucial to the success of the demonstration was how we came apart, using eye-contact to ensure that both of us withdrew the force together. This was then passed around the circle a couple of times, with greater general success the second time. The children improved both their ability to channel their energy, find or maintain eye-contact and to come apart respectfully. I repeated this movement over several sessions, with noticeable improvements among the children in concentration, ability to channel energy and placing of the whole body.

So, what were the benefits of these particular movement experiences for the children, some of whom had demonstrated anti-social playground behaviours? The benefits were: relationships built through shared experiences, not only with immediate partners, but also with the larger group; and an increased body knowledge and sense of centre – particularly apparent in some of the children. Legitimately being allowed actually to push someone with a lot of strength – an activity usually frowned on in the playground – was much enjoyed. However, added to this was the responsibility of caring for their partner when breaking out of the 'against' relationship. This changed a strong 'against' relationship into a 'caring' one, giving the children a chance to demonstrate that they, who were usually cared for, were capable of behaving in a caring manner. The activity provided them with an opportunity to develop and grow socially and to increase in self-esteem.

Sherborne described in her book how children with learning disabilities often do not seem to possess a keen sense of centre. The movement experiences above, with appropriate support from staff, appeared to help several of the children in the groups to develop an ability to push from their centre. They constructively channelled the energy of certain members of the class, who could be praised for being both strong and gentle at the same time. One particular boy, who was large for his age, discovered how to achieve success with these activities despite working with the smallest and lightest boy in the class.

We then moved onto Sherborne's 'back-to-back slides'. This is another 'with' movement experience, but this time the children were organised in pairs sitting back-to-back. This movement develops awareness of self and others, not only of the immediate partner, but also of all the other partnerships operating in the room. One child has their legs outstretched and their hands in their lap, whilst the other child pushes against their back and, thus, slides them across the floor. The children develop an increased sense of body awareness, especially of their backs plus hips and legs as these slide along the ground. The pusher uses their feet and hands against the floor, and sometimes turns round and pushes with other body parts. All of this effort confirms a knowledge of these body parts, and thus increases a sense of self. Sometimes a little help is needed to support the child who is learning how to push. The care-giver working with them can praise when the tiniest pushing movement is detected, and the partner can oblige by moving sufficiently far for the pusher to gain a sense of pushing. There is much laughter when various partnerships collide or miss each other. In my experience, this is a very social exercise and great fun for everyone involved.

The creative part of the sessions proved to be very popular with the children in the two groups. I divided the children into groups – between two and four children with a member of staff. The task was for each member of the group to choose their favourite movement from the session, teach it to the other members of the group, and then for the group to join these favourite movements together to make a short dance. (In the case of pairs, two favourite movements each were needed – not much of a problem for the more able child.) Variations of 'pass the touch' frequently appeared, as did the pushing in various forms. Another favourite was 'tail spins', where children sat on the floor and span round, sometimes deliberately falling over and rolling up again.

All these SDM movement experiences addressed these children's need to channel their energy more positively, to be involved physically with other children without being aggressive, and, through this, to develop self-esteem. The staff commented on how well the children were behaving together, and, in particular, how well they could work together in pairs. I, having nothing to compare progress with, just took the sessions at face value, and noted the progression through the activities, who could do what, and thought about how I could help each child to develop their understanding of their body and have a good time dancing. Nevertheless, the staff were impressed with the development of the children's social skills within this series of the classes. I do not know whether playground behaviour has improved, but this insight gave impetus to good work by the children.

So why do I use SDM? Well – because it appears to work. The philosophy of 'developing relationships' and 'being at home in our bodies' through movement experiences is central to my work as a community dance worker. My work also needs to be thoroughly enjoyable for all participants. Movement experiences can be presented in a way that is achievable for participants, and in such a way that the participants realise that they are achievable – both personally and through feedback from others. They gradually develop a good sense of centre, which is physically satisfying, and movement experiences with a partner enable people to feel connected to others and just as importantly to themselves. I see both of these as basic human needs – to feel connected to ourselves and to others.

I believe that we are all able to enjoy aesthetic experiences, and that we are all creative in some way. I aim to provide the best possible dance experiences for the people I am privileged to work with, and I find that the foundation and philosophy of SDM enables me to do this more effectively.

References

Csikszentmihalyi, M. (1992) *Flow: The psychology of happiness.* London: Ryder.

Sherborn, V. (2001) *Developmental Movement for Children: Mainstream, special needs and pre-school* (2nd edn). London: Worth Publishing.

Smith-Autard, J.M. (1994) *The Art of Dance in Education.* London: Black.

SDM and Therapy – a Team Approach
Danny Dossche and Ingeborg Vandamme (Physiotherapists), Ilse Bontinck and Nathalie Vanassche (Occupational Therapists), and Marleen Van Rentergem and Kurt Fierens (Speech and Language Therapists)

In this section, we would like to describe and explain our work with SDM in therapeutics in a 'readaptation centre' in Deinze, Belgium.

We work with developmentally delayed children, aged between three months and six years, with varying needs. The children have mental, emotional, physical and/or behavioural difficulties. We work in multidisciplinary teams, each consisting of a speech and language therapist, a physiotherapist and an occupational therapist, under the supervision of a psychologist and a paediatric doctor. Therapy is adapted to the needs of every child and can be given individually or in small groups of four children. The children come to the Centre for one and a half hours, three times a week. The therapists give them specific individual therapy, and, once a week, there is an SDM session with the children and therapists coming together as a group.

Together with the long-term aims, short-term goals are regularly discussed, re-assessed and evaluated by the team, in deliberation with the parents of the child.

In the course of working with these young children with developmental delay, we had felt the need for a transdisciplinary setting, in addition to the individual therapeutic sessions. In the transdisciplinary setting, every member of the team was involved holistically with the child with special needs. Every therapist had a certain knowledge of the work of his colleagues, and therefore was able to work together with them, in the same room, with the same group of children, implementing the therapies in the same developmental direction. Every member of the team had full responsibility for the whole development of the child. These children are at very early stages of development, and so react very globally, and it is up to us as therapists to understand the child and guide him in his process of development.

For several years, we worked in our transdisciplinary team with small groups of children in so-called 'social-communicative' groups. Professionals from different therapeutic disciplines worked closely together in delivering their therapy for each child. Our work with each child was based on the development of a basic trust in themselves and in their environment. We 'played' together in a room, with only ourselves and the children, without any material: rolling, sliding, rocking, jumping, running – just being together.

We experienced that, after a while, the children loved to play with us, and they took the initiative in communication. In the beginning, communication was mostly non-verbal; later on, or with the older children, verbal exchanges took place. The children experimented with new games – they challenged us! These children with varying needs, with developmental difficulties, taught *us* how to play, how to enjoy being together as equal partners with respect for each other. These little people, at very early stages of development, opened themselves up to their environment and went to the environment for new discoveries.

At that time, we heard about SDM. It was magnificent to recognise the basic philosophy of SDM as the thing we were looking for. At last, we had found a base to our work, and we could translate our goals into SDM terms.

As well as having the same basic philosophy and the same therapeutic direction, every team member has his own qualifications and, within the total therapeutic programme of the child, brings his own expertise. Currently, we still have our specific, individual, therapeutic programme for each child – which can also include individual SDM when a child is not able yet to join in the group – and, on a weekly basis, we have an SDM hour with groups of children with various developmental needs.

Our whole therapeutic team has attained Level 3 in SDM training – and, in one of the multidisciplinary teams, which consists of a speech and language therapist, an occupational therapist and a physiotherapist, all are qualified international course leaders in SDM. As a team of international course leaders, we often organise 'basic' (Levels 1 and 2) courses or we are asked by different institutions to give courses on SDM. The participants are mostly therapists (physio-, occupational and speech), but also many psychologists, nurses, educators, nursery care-givers and teachers are interested in the courses, and enthusiastic to use SDM in their daily work.

1. Physiotherapy for young children with developmental delay or disturbance (motor problems)

Working as physiotherapists with young children means that we have to help these children to develop their motor skills as well as possible. The physical problems that they may have (e.g. myasthenia, contractures, postural problems, etc.) can disturb this development and therefore must be treated through specific physiotherapeutic treatment. But this treatment on its own is not enough!

If we observe children with a typical locomotor development, it is obvious that they move a lot, that they enjoy moving, that they move fluently, and that there is a lot of variation in their movement. They exercise their new motor skills by doing them over and over again, just because moving is fun! Children with a developmental delay or disturbance are often rather passive and do not have the drive to search for new things to learn and discover. Some are, on the contrary, over-active. They move a lot, move quickly, but do not take the time to learn about the things they meet.

All parents are concerned about the development of their children. The motor development is the most striking part of young children's progression and that is why parents check whether their child reaches the motor milestones at the right time. If a child fails to sit, crawl, stand or walk at the expected age, parents are alarmed that something could be wrong. The delay in their child's motor development is often the reason that parents bring their children for examination and treatment. The parents then expect us to teach their children new motor skills – but movement therapy can be much more!

If we want a child to learn to move in a better way, it is very important to teach this child that moving is fun. That way, the child's 'need to move' will grow, he will move more without anyone asking him to do so, and will therefore practise his newly gained motor skills, and use them when not in therapy. If we succeed in this, we have obtained our first requirement – that 'they move…and they enjoy it!'

There are several reasons why we think that Sherborne's method can be very useful in helping us reach this goal:

- The relationship between the child and the therapist is an equal-partner relationship. It is not always the therapist who teaches something to the child, but both partners share the movement experiences. They play together, doing enjoyable movement activities. The child also can initiate the next movement. This can stimulate his feeling of competence.

- Feeling his body against another (therapist or other partner) will make the child more conscious of his own body. He will learn what his possibilities and restrictions are, and therefore feel more confident to try new movements.

- Having a lot of body-contact can help us in observing the body language of the child and help us to react in a sensitive/responsive way. Muscle tension can give us a lot of information about the child – for example, if he is in pain, if he dislikes touch, etc. Especially for children who do not have the opportunity to communicate using language, this body-contact, in addition to eye-contact, is very important.

- The atmosphere of the whole group can motivate the children enormously. Seeing children amusing themselves with movement games can be a reason to join in. We never have to coerce them to do this. Also, for children with a learning disability, it is a good way to invite them to play with the group. Sometimes they do not understand a verbal task, but now they can imitate the others.

- We do not insist on a perfect quality for the children's movements. We can respect them within their own possibilities and their own restrictions. They can work at their own level to reach their goals, and so they feel themselves respected, which results in them having more trust in their own potential. Their self-confidence will grow and that will stimulate them to explore.

With SDM, we just have to acknowledge that we have found a perfect symbiosis between our specific motor aims and our aim that the children enjoy the movement. However, with children who have cerebral palsy, we have to use our knowledge about the specific motor problem, and therefore we are very careful to avoid some contra-indicated activities.

As physiotherapists, we are very familiar with the words 'psychomotor therapy'. This is a treatment which always starts from 'corporeal movement', and which influences systematically the personality of the child in a positive way. In the personality of the child, we always see three interdependent components: motor cognition, motor control and social effectiveness. Sherborne's approach can help us to reach the child in each of these components and to have a positive influence on them. In all of these areas, we can obtain some good results using Sherborne's ideas.

Motor Control
The playing of movement games includes the training of different motor skills (e.g. rolling, crawling, running, etc.). Through SDM, these skills improve. If we are lucky enough to work in a 1:1 relationship, we can directly help the child if he has some problems. As physiotherapists, we are convinced of the importance of the muscle tone. Having good muscle tone is one of the main pillars of our motor development. With SDM, we have a lot of opportunities to work on it. Laban's words, 'energy' and 'flow', suit perfectly in this context. We start by making the child conscious of his centre, and then try to build up muscle tone there. This is not only necessary in order to have a good connection between the trunk and the limbs, but is also very important in the development of self-awareness. A strong centre makes the child more conscious of himself and his place in this world – it gives him the inner motivation to move and so to be able to develop.

Motor Cognition
Training the motor cognition aspect is not always our first and primary intention when we are doing SDM, but that does not mean that SDM has no effect on it. Often we see that children, without being conscious of it, develop and improve in this respect. Their concentration increases over the several sessions. Working in a sensitive/responsive way results in a joint attention. SDM also stimulates them in exploring their personal space and the space around them. They explore concepts such as 'under', 'up', 'fast', etc. If we name the movement qualities as they experience them, it will surely help them afterwards to use the right words in their verbal communication.

Social Effectiveness
The importance of this component is well-known to SDM practitioners. We work on it by using the three different kinds of relationships described by Sherborne.

In a **'with' relationship**, we 'take care of' our child, and we give him the physical and emotional security he needs to become more confident. A good 'together/shared' relationship ensures that both partners feel equally important. Together we can do it, so we both have to do the best we can!

In an **'against' relationship**, the child can test his own strength against that of the older partner. If the older partner adjusts to the strength of the child, the child is encouraged to use all the energy he has and will experience success. 'Emotional stability', 'security' and 'confidence' are some of the key words in psychomotor development, as they are in SDM.

Conclusion

These are only a few examples of how SDM can support us in stimulating the psychomotor development. Working with Sherborne's approach in therapy is very interesting. It offers us a lot of opportunities in our work as physiotherapists.

Whatever their difficulty is, we have the same aims for all our children. Whether the client is a child who has cerebral palsy, Down's syndrome, ASD or hyperactivity, it is our task to be creative to discover their special needs and to improve their quality of life. Therefore it is not only their movement that is important, but we also have to take into account their whole personality. This will not only change our clients (both children and adults) – it can even help our own development. In our busy, 21st-century life, sometimes we neglect our own bodies and ignore the value of them!

2. Occupational Therapy for Babies, Toddlers and Infants with Varying Developmental Delay

As occupational therapists (OTs), we are part of the multidisciplinary team, and our work focuses on different aspects of the total development of the child. In our therapeutic setting, the OT is the 'in-between' link between the physiotherapist and the speech and language therapist. The OT conducts the child towards independence in his physical, psychological and social-emotional life in their daily business, leaning backwards on the therapy of the physiotherapist and leading forwards to the therapy of the speech and language therapist.

The OT's aims in a therapeutic setting focus on the development of:

- Fine motor praxis: manipulation skills, eye–motor co-ordination, bimanual co-ordination, etc.
- Visual perception: visual attention, object permanency, object constancy, figure–ground perception, visual memory, etc.
- Activities of daily living: dressing, personal hygiene, etc.
- Psychomotricity: exploration of the environment, organisation and structuring of the nearby surroundings, projection of space in different dimensions and directions, motivation and an inner drive to experiment
- Complex tasks: table-based, learning skills – sorting, drawing, counting.

In our therapy, we have to start out from a base point of psychological well-being, where the child has a positive self-esteem and is ready to look outward to the environment and the others around. Out of this basic feeling, we will be able to guide the child's playing.

The child spends most of his daily life playing, and he has to develop all his skills out of his experiences in play. The basic requirements for achieving independence come out of playing. Children with developmental delay do not learn typically. As OTs, we help them to focus their attention and to increase their skills by adapting their play to their own levels of competence.

Before we can start working with different kinds of materials, it is necessary that the child learns to play with us, without material, focusing his attention on himself and the therapist. It is in this very early stage of individual OT guidance that we introduce SDM. We use SDM to become an equal partner with the child in a beneficial 'playing' environment. The child builds up confidence in us; he builds up trust in us, and he learns that we will not let him down, or let him fail. To guide the child to new experiences, it is our task as OTs to be sure that the child is ready to try out and to reach for new experiences – for himself, from within himself, out of his own inner motivation and not because we ask him to do so. As OTs, we observe the children and anticipate their next step forward.

Playing is a real voyage of discovery; it is the great adventure of life, where a child can feel safe and sure. The safety of the play stimulates the self-confidence of the child. Furthermore, by bringing the challenge of the play up to the developmental level of the child, he gets the experience of success and builds up a positive self-esteem, which in turn leads to independence. This gives the child the possibility of broadening his competency and his own functional independence. This accords with how Sherborne saw the development of the child – as growing towards freedom and autonomy within the borders of personal talents and possibilities.

With very young children (aged 0–2 years), SDM is an answer to their needs at Piaget's 'sensory motor' developmental stage. The young child's cognitive development is characterised by their motor reactions to sensorial input. At this stage, the sensorial perception is dominant, and the child learns to know his body, step by step. All of his daily life is focused on discovery and examination of himself and the surroundings, including the people he meets. Associated with the child's physical development, we see psychological development – the social-emotional development, the attention and concentration of the child. We have to be aware how the child feels and how he reacts or even if he will react at all to the stimulus.

Both developmental areas – physical and psychological – are stimulated by playing. By playing, we use the only way a child is able to learn, discover and experience. At this stage, there is not much language, and children scout around in the environment and get to know themselves by moving or by being moved.

SDM helps the child become a less egocentric person and to grow towards being a purposeful explorer.

In terms of SDM, we speak about all movement experiences where we try to stimulate the child within his personal abilities by cradling, containing, sliding, by using different movement qualities in terms of time and energy, and by moving in different directions and with different body parts. We start in all kinds of 'with' relationships, where we support the child before he becomes aware of himself and is able to move by himself and become aware of his surroundings and other people. We do not hesitate to bring very young children together in the same room, each of them with their own care-giver, working alongside each other until they are able to 'see' the others and start working together more and more.

When a child feels confident enough, we can bring him materials with which he can explore new experiences using his body and his developing spatial awareness. When the OT introduces the right toys at the right moment, the child is stimulated to continue his voyage of discovery because he is confronted with a challenge that is adjusted to his developmental level. It is at this moment that the OT changes from his direct use of SDM as a therapeutic tool to applying the basic philosophy of SDM as guidance principle in other activities.

When we use material to stimulate the child in the generally accepted OT context, or whenever the child is ready for this 'material' aspect of our therapeutic approach, we do not forget the principles we used in SDM. We invite the child to be creative, to take initiative, and we stay and play together with the child. It is still very important that the child feels safe and sure, feels confident and trusted.

We keep contact with the child – doing the same thing at the same place in the same time. We give the child positive experiences and help him to discover and use his own potential, to build up a positive self-esteem. The child goes on playing, but learns now to pay attention to objects and makes the transition from Piaget's early sensorimotor stage to a more pre-operational stage. At this stage (age 2–7 years), the child is able to make better sense of and organise his surroundings, and language also helps him to regulate the world around by naming objects. In this period, the social factor is also very important. The child takes into account not only material and objects, but he is also in communication with the partner providing the material. The child builds up creativity and enjoys being busy.

SDM is, for the OT, not only a therapeutic medium, but also a basic philosophy with which to support and maintain the therapy.

3. The Speech and Language Therapist

In speech and language therapy, we have five important goals:

- Speech (how to pronounce different vocals, consonants, etc.)
- Semantics (the meaning of words)
- Grammatics (making new words)
- Syntaxis (combining words)
- Pragmatics (the use of language in communication).

The use of language within relationships with others is, for us as speech and language therapists, the most important link to Sherborne's philosophy.

Pragmatics involves three major aspects:

- Communicative intentions
- Organisation of the discourse
- Presupposition.

When we communicate, there is always a *context*. If the context changes, the same sentence can have a totally different meaning. The context influences these three important communication aspects: communicative intentions, presupposition and social organisation of the discourse.

To influence the context, we do not push the children into a passive or static role. We concentrate on the subjects that the children bring (verbal and/or non-verbal intentions). We do not only work with pictures, but also with real objects, toys, actions, and even without any material (actions, movement, rhythm). We search for an activity that matches with the specific needs of the children so we can obtain a natural, child-focused conversation.

Often speech and language therapy starts with children who are not aware of their own communicative signals; they are 'not looking at', 'not reaching for', etc. For the child and adult, the **communicative intentions** are not always obvious. In therapy, we try to reach seven important communicative intentions (Roth and Speakman, 1984). The lowest level is non-verbal and gestural. This gives way to a combination of non-verbal with verbal intention, and to the final level: verbal communicative intentions.

The first communicative intention is making the others pay attention to you, to things that happen, to objects or to other persons. Request follows: request for objects, for action, for information. Greeting is another important intention, followed by giving something to another. Protesting and aborting are intentions that can be easily stimulated, and the last two are answering (confirming) and informing. We try to stimulate these intentions in a joint action or joint attention, and often we give some teasing or blocking tasks (e.g. letting a child try to open a door that cannot be opened, keeping the last puzzle piece in our own hand, etc.). In SDM sessions, there are many opportunities to enhance communicative intention: e.g. 'Look there', reaching hands, asking for help, 'high fives' as a greeting, 'Let me out' (when an adult holds the child firmly), 'enjoying being rolled over' and asking for more – 'once more'.

The second aspect of pragmatics is learning the rules of conversation, the **social organisation of the discourse**. We start with a relationship between the therapist and the child, progress to a child–child relationship, and culminate in a child–stranger relationship. 'Turn-taking' is the central phrase: we try to share the same level of communication, so we can agree or disagree about a subject. Important aspects are, for example, an appropriate way to greet each other, maintain a conversation, discover or use the non-verbal signs in conversation – distance between speaker and listener, facial expressions, eye-contact, etc. In SDM sessions, we practise turn-taking many times: greeting sessions on the floor; saying, 'Hello,' to everybody in the room, with your hands, feet, etc.; sharing a 'see-saw'. All these are aspects of Sherborne's relationship play.

The third goal is **presupposition**: adapting your language to the needs or expectations of the listener. Around the age of four, children are developing a theory of mind. They can convey mental states (thoughts, emotions, wishes) to themselves and others, and they have the ability to anticipate these states. Children with a mental age below four years can be stimulated to develop the basic foundations of theory of mind. Important aspects are: the stimulation of joint action, joint attention and imitation (oral–facial, body gestures, vocal–verbal, object manipulation). Discovery and differentiation of the basic feelings (happy, angry, afraid and sad) are very nice to open a conversation with and to stimulate presupposition. In relationship play, partners observe mental states, and adapt their behaviour through the imitation of each other's movements with arms, hands, head (e.g. through playing 'Mirror', etc.). As Rudolf Laban writes:

> *Movement is first and fundamental in what comes forth from a human being as an expression of his intentions and experiences.*

In the area of speech and language, intentional communication takes a lot of our interest and attention. Intentional communication is necessary when we relate to other people. This communication can be verbal or non-verbal.

Non-verbal communication is very useful when we share emotions, experiences and information with others. It is present in everyone from their first day of life, but initially it is not intentional. The crying baby brings the adult into action: we try to comfort the baby as if he was really asking for it. When a baby is satisfied and happy, one can observe its state by looking to the body movements and signals. We respond to the baby's actions as if they were signs of intentional communicating instead of reflexive acts.

By eight weeks, approximately, social interaction and turn-taking, initiated by the adult, begin when the adult and the baby are smiling at one another face-to-face and making cooing sounds. By six or seven months, the infant is babbling and the social interaction has improved a lot. You can have long 'conversations' making sounds back and forth to each other. About nine months, the infant communicates intentionally and becomes very sociable. The interaction with the adult is based on intentionality and reciprocity. The child makes requests, gets your attention, can show you things and greet you by using conventional gestures and sounds as if they were words. A few months later, the code of spoken language is 'cracked'.

Learning language takes place during everyday, fun **interactions** with adults and peers. Children need to participate actively in these interactions in order to learn to communicate and use language. They need our help and **information** as conversation partners in order to learn the rules of interaction and conversation.

A good conversation partner is, for example, able to:

- Initiate interaction or respond when others initiate
- Take a turn at the appropriate time
- Give the partner a chance to take a turn
- Give attention to the partner
- Continue the interaction or conversation by taking additional turns on the topic
- Send clear messages
- Clear up misunderstandings
- Stick to the subject
- Initiate a new topic when appropriate.

In terms of SDM, these qualities are the very same when we speak of good partnership in an SDM session.

As speech and language therapists, we need to create opportunities for the children to interact, and we have to use strategies that help them learn the rules of interaction and conversation. Learning language is a process in which the therapist and the child are both participating and learning from one another. Interaction routines, such as feeding, washing and playing, are crucial in this process of learning. The situation in the routine is meaningful for both partners, and language can grow out of this meaningful and repeated context. Of course, a lot of turn-taking together is needed to build the interaction and communication. That is where conversations take place!

Our role is more than just modelling language. We have to try to understand the child, and the child must be able to understand us. Our interaction style must be very sensitive and responsive. We have to wait, observe and listen carefully so we can see the initiations of the child, and we can give an adequate response. By being with a responsive therapist, the child can gain a sense of pleasure from communication, the desire to initiate, and last, but not least, more opportunities to learn language.

In playing together, we learn that we do not need a lot of toys or objects to have a good interaction or conversation. Especially with babies, infants or toddlers, or with people at a lower-than-typical stage of language development, it is appropriate to work with a minimal provision of objects. Dividing your attention between your conversation partner and a toy can be too difficult at an early developmental stage.

In Dent's study (1993), we can read that SDM is a good context for playing with children with developmental delay. They can gain social experiences to stimulate the sense of body self and subjective self. According to the theory of Stern, these senses of self are basic to the development of the sense of symbolic self in which the use of language is the most important ability.

'Sense of self' has been conceptualised as having subjective and objective features and is considered to have evolved out of physical and psychological structures as well as from experiences within the context of a relationship with a significant other (Dent, 1993). When we think of goals in therapy when dealing with children or adults in the early stages of language development, we can reach for, for example, mutual focus of attention on a partner in interaction, intentional communication, turn-taking and imitation.

SDM is a very good way of playing together and can be built up as a play routine, where the partners know the context and where communication and conversation can take place with or without words. Practising SDM in an appropriate way is like having a good conversation, where therapist and child can send messages as equal partners, focusing on one another, taking equal turns together within a mutual context (moving together), staying with this context and being true and genuine to each other. The goals to reach for in therapy can be easily realised using SDM as a medium, especially when starting at the non-verbal level. Spoken language can be gradually introduced and generated when appropriate. Then real conversations can begin whilst partners are moving together.

General Bibliography and References

Ayres, A.J. (1975) *Southern California Sensory Integration Test* (SCSIT). Los Angeles: Western Psychological Services.
Dent, C. (1993) Play with and without objects: effects on the sense of self of the child with Down's syndrome. Calgary: University of Calgary. (Unpublished MD thesis)
Lefebvre, J.J. (1974) *Information Optimale*. Montreal, Canada: Conceptions 2001 Inc.
Manolson, A. (1985) *It Takes Two to Talk*. Toronto, Canada: The Hanen Program.
Piaget J.J. (1969) *The Psychology of the Child*. New York: Basic Books.
Roth, F. and Speakman, N. (1984) 'Assessing the pragmatic ability of children: part 1. organizational framework and assessment parameters', *Journal of Speech and Hearing Disorders*, 49, 2–11.
Schaerlaeckens, A.M. and Gillis, S. (1987) *De Taalverwerving van Het Kind*. Groningen, Netherlands: Wolters-Noordhoff.
Sherborne, V. (2001) *Developmental Movement for Children: Mainstream, special needs and pre-school* (2nd edn). London: Worth Publishing.
Stern, D.N. (1985) *The Interpersonal World of the Infant*. New York: Basic Books.
Weizman, E. (1992) *Learning Language and Loving It*. Toronto, Canada: The Hanen Program.

A Physiotherapist's view of Sherborne Developmental Movement
Chris Handley

I would like to share my experiences of using SDM after several colleagues and I attended an introductory course. For many years, I have worked with children with a wide range of difficulties, and I moved to a school for children with learning disabilities in Staffordshire in 1997. It was here that my interest in 'Sherborne' began.

The school is for children, aged 3–18 years, with learning difficulties. Some of these children have profound motor and learning difficulties, and I found this group particularly difficult to motivate. They often disliked being handled and moved – by anyone, not just the physiotherapy staff. As such young people become bigger and heavier, it presents more of a problem.

It has been my experience that a number of treatment principles can complement each other, no one method being the answer for any child. I feel that 'Sherborne' supports and enriches both Conductive and Bobath systems.

After observing Sherborne methods being used with early years children, I began to realise a lot of the basic principles fitted in with what I was trying to achieve. My main problem was enabling children to experience more typical activity in response to therapeutic handling. Bringing children into an SDM-based movement group helped me to facilitate, motivate and give sensations of movement.

SDM contributes to developing body and spatial awareness, an important skill requirement in other methods of treatment. In conductive education, a stable base and hands, hips and knees are key areas. In Bobath theory, for typical movement to be learned, a child must be able to perform movements for themselves and be motivated to succeed. What better way than having fun in a group with all your friends?

Within the group setting, the physiotherapist can contribute her knowledge and respond to the other members of the team involved with each child. Group working is an important means by which the physiotherapist can become part of the team – not only with education staff, but also with the carers, parents and, most importantly, with the child.

The parents I have worked with have been amazed at the communication and enjoyment of movement their children are capable of. They are able to use some of the activities at home to play with their child and encourage tone-inhibiting positions. Parents are much more likely to do this if they and their children are enjoying the experience. It is not just another task that they, as carers, have to perform in an already hectic schedule.

At present, I am working with a group of nursery-aged children to develop good relationships and enjoyment of movement. I also support education staff working with older children. In recognising how SDM is able to complement other physiotherapy concepts, I hope to make possible improvements in handling and activity for children who, in the past, have experienced difficulties in these areas

Within our Physiotherapy Peer Support Group, we hope to extend the integration of the Sherborne concepts, and include children attending other schools in the area.

CHAPTER 6
Sherborne Developmental Movement in Education

In this chapter, we will be working entirely in the field of education, as this is the area in which Sherborne developed her ideas, and where Sherborne Developmental Movement (SDM) is still most widely used in the UK.

It would appear that Sherborne came to use her ideas with children with special needs almost by accident! In her book, she describes how she first introduced her ideas with students who were being trained to teach children with severe learning difficulties, with a view to making them feel secure within the group, using partner and group activities. She wrote:

> *To my surprise, the students went on to introduce some of the partner activities to the children with severe learning difficulties, with some success, and it became clear to me that children too could relate to these kinds of activities.* (Sherborne, 2001, p. xiii)*

The 'children' to whom Sherborne referred were, in the main, ambulant – some had quite skilful physical ability, and some had emotional and behavioural difficulties, in many cases combined with a lot of energy! They mostly attended special schools in either the community or the large institutions of the time. It was with this group of children that Sherborne continued to develop and hone her ideas. This process continued over the subsequent years, with her ideas continuing to be used in special education after it became part of the national education system in the early 1970s. (Previously, the 'education' of children with severe learning difficulties had been the responsibility of the health authorities.)

However, with the introduction of the National Curriculum, the use of SDM in special schools went into a noticeable decline. Where did 'Sherborne' fit into a new, apparently very strict and demanding scheme of things? It didn't have a 'label', which would have allowed it to slot easily into the requirements for Physical Education (PE) or the 'core subjects'. Demands on teachers to comply and meet many and diverse requirements subjected them to an almost overwhelming amount of re-thinking and re-planning of timetables and classroom activities. Understandably, there just was not time or room for something that really did not appear to fit in anywhere!

But there was a positive side to this trend. Teachers of pupils with profound and multiple learning difficulties started to ask how their children could access the National Curriculum. Here SDM was able to provide some of the answers in terms of the early communication, sensory experiences and body awareness required within Key Stage 1 for the core subjects, and, on the majority of our courses, I was beginning to notice that there was a strong element of interest focused on the use of SDM with pupils and students with profound and multiple learning difficulties.

Whilst being very pleased with, and supportive of, this growing trend, I was also becoming very concerned about the decline of the work with the more physically able children and young people. I felt that some way needed to be found to re-establish interest in using Sherborne's approach among this group. Having used her ideas in my own teaching with pupils with severe learning difficulties and profound and multiple learning difficulties over a considerable number of years, I personally had no doubts about its appropriateness and benefits for the children with whom I worked, in terms of both their learning experiences and personal development. After some deliberation, I came to the conclusion that the Sherborne philosophy that 'we meet the participants where they are' must also be true for teachers! We had to 'meet them where *they* were' – within the National Curriculum requirements.

When the National Curriculum was introduced in its original form, it required a great deal of ingenuity to find ways of enabling access for our pupils with severe learning difficulties and profound and multiple learning difficulties, but, even at that early stage, it was possible with some degree of 'lateral and innovative thinking' to slot some of Sherborne's ideas into aspects of the early key stages. Since the initial introduction, however, a great deal of consideration has been given to extending the document in order to make it far more accessible to pupils across the entire spectrum of special needs, with the result that, reading through the present Qualifications and Curriculum Authority (QCA) guidelines for the core subjects of English, Mathematics and Science, and for Physical Education (PE) and Personal, Social and Health Education (PSHE) and Citizenship, it becomes apparent that there are many different ways in which SDM can very meaningfully support access to the curriculum for our pupils with severe and multiple learning difficulties.

The following tables, under each of the subject headings, cross-reference many of the QCA 'Opportunities and activities' and 'Performance descriptions' with relevant SDM activities. The page numbers in the tables refer to QCA subject guidelines.

English

QCA GUIDELINES	SDM
Responding to pupils' needs (p. 4) 'Learning English encompasses all aspects of communication – non-verbal, verbal and written.'	**Communication** is a fundamental aspect of SDM at *all* times. Participants are encouraged to express/indicate how they feel about the activities, their preferences, likes and dislikes. There is a continual dialogue between everyone taking part in the session, albeit through various means – verbal exchange, body language, eye-contact, facial expression or gesture.
Speaking and listening (p. 5) 'Communication may include the use of whole-body movements, gesture.'	Work on **space** includes establishing 'personal space' – that being space *immediately* in front, behind, to each side, above, below – sometimes **sharing** it with another person or group of people by making movements in which hands or feet are touching; sometimes **defending** it by pushing 'against' another person and keeping them at a distance, in a way that is assertive, but not aggressive.
Speaking (p. 5.) '…encourage pupils to express their likes, dislikes, feelings…through a range of communicative movements and gestures.'	Developing an awareness of Laban's 'movement qualities' – in terms of movements which are heavy/light, fast/slow, in straight/flexible lines, tight and 'bound'/very 'free' – and learning to incorporate these varying qualities into our movements greatly extends our movement vocabulary and therefore our ability to communicate our feelings through body language and gesture.
Listening and responding (p. 6) 'It is important to develop the ability to…maintain and develop concentration.'	Sherborne's 'against' relationship experiences require us to test our strength against the resistance of another person. In order to be able to do this successfully, we have to be able to focus and direct energy on the task in hand. We 'feel' what it is like to direct attention, to stay on task and to concentrate. 'Shared' balance activities require us to focus attention and to concentrate on our partner.
Key Stage 1 (p. 13) '…focus may be on giving pupils opportunities to…work in role'	Intrinsic in Sherborne's 'with/caring' relationship activities are two distinct roles: that of the person who is being looked after/cared for, and that of the person who is responsible for that person's well-being and feeling of security.

Indications from the above table suggest that SDM can mostly support access to the English curriculum in the area of 'communication', not only through the use of verbal communication, but also in terms of developing the confidence to communicate through the use of gesture and body language. Communication opens the way to consideration and enquiry as to how I feel about myself and how I feel about others. Given appropriate opportunities at Key Stage 4, the QCA guidelines suggest that:

> *Pupils are enabled to develop, maintain and consolidate their communication skills in preparation for adult life.* (p. 26)

On one of our SDM courses, one participant remarked:

> *Sherborne Developmental Movement is like a microcosm of life – it gives us the opportunity to explore many of life's experiences in a non-threatening non-judgemental way.*

Mathematics

QCA GUIDELINES	SDM
Modifying the Mathematics programme of study (p. 5) **Shape, space and measures** '…the main focus will be to build on the way pupils respond to similarities and differences, *for example, in position, movement, size, weight…*' (p. 6) 'Teaching shape, space…across the key stages can help pupils to: …develop their awareness of position, distance, movement and direction… '…acquire mathematical language associated with shape, space…'	Work on spatial concepts focuses on 'where we are in space/relative positions in space'. Discussions centre around *'How can I tell the difference between "in front" and "behind"?', ' Is "on" the same as "over" – if not, why is it different?', 'How can I help my partner to understand the meaning of "on", "under", "through"?'* In its very simplest terms, by just resting my hand **on** your head, or, in a more advanced way, by supporting my partner **on** my back/knees. By making a shape with our bodies, which we can travel **through**, etc. All of these spatial considerations can be explored through movement experiences, which *must* be accompanied by the **appropriate language** to describe precisely what is happening. Much of Sherborne's 'body awareness' work, again accompanied by **appropriate language**, can focus the attention on body posture, size and shape. For example, in 'awareness of centres', the focus is on staying curled up, very **small and tight**, but in preparation for that activity, in order for us to experience the contrast, we can make body shapes, which are very **big**. In 'open and closed rolling', the body is alternately **long and short**, and we can also make body shapes, which help us to feel **wide and narrow, high and low**. Space can also be explored by 'running, jumping **high,** landing, tumbling and rolling into **low** space on the floor'.

Although the above table indicates very clearly that SDM can most meaningfully support access to the National Curriculum in the areas of shape, space and direction, as in every subject there are always many opportunities for the development of mathematical skills such as:

- number
- size of groups working together
- sequences of movements – e.g. spin on hips/tumble/roll/spin on hips…etc. (Key Stage 1, p. 8)
- direction – travelling backwards, forwards, sideways.

Communicating through Movement

Science

QCA GUIDELINES	SDM
Life processes and living things (p. 6) 'Knowledge and understanding of humans…starts with pupils' awareness of themselves, *for example, body awareness and self awareness*, and, at first, relates to personal experience, *for example… experiencing movement, exploring their own body parts…*'	Through her observations and experiences one of the main conclusions which Sherborne arrived at, was that *'children need to feel at home in their own body…'** therefore the development of good body awareness and self-image became one of the prime objectives of her work. She wrote on it in considerable detail in her book, in which she describes numerous activities designed to increase body awareness in terms of naming body parts and becoming aware of how they work, both separately and in a co-ordinated way, giving children the ability to move with confidence within their individual physical abilities.
Physical processes **Forces and motion** (p. 8) 'Knowledge and understanding of forces and motion starts by experiencing a range of movements followed by feeling and anticipating their effects…Teaching this aspect …can help pupils to: • make movement happen by applying a force • recognise that when things speed up, slow down or change direction or shape, there is a cause, *for example a push or pull.*'	Many of Sherborne's relationship activities require the application of force. For example, the 'against' relationship activities require us to test our strength against that of our partner, either by, for example, **pushing** against them to 'destabilise the rock' or **pulling** against them to 'unwrap the parcel'. The 'with' relationship activity, 'sliding', involves one partner giving the other a slide by **pulling** him along the floor by the ankles or hands. *'Can you give your partner a **fast** slide? Now give your partner a **slow** slide. Which took the most **energy**?'* Individual sliding on stomachs/backs offers the opportunity to discuss force and direction. *'When we **pull** with our hands, which direction do we go in? When we **push** with our hands we go…?*
Key Stage 1 (p. 10) 'The focus of teaching science at Key Stage 1 may be on giving pupils the opportunity to: • engage in practical activities and investigations that extend their awareness and understanding of themselves, *for example, body awareness and self-awareness.*'	See above for 'body awareness'. Part of 'self-awareness' is development of our knowledge concerning our *ability* to move and the *way* in which we move. SDM gives us the opportunity to investigate and explore different ways of moving, and to decide from those experiences which of those ways is most beneficial and comfortable for us as individuals (see Chapter 4).
Key Stage 2 (p. 16) **Forces** 'Pupils explore and investigate movement, pushing and pulling. They may: • experience a variety of different movements, *for example being rocked and rolled in a safe and comfortable context…* • move their bodies by being supported or pushed at different speeds and in different directions'	One of Sherborne's 'whole body' experiences is 'rolling' either individually, or working with a partner in a 'caring/with' relationship activity. In this case the person being rolled can either be **pulled** and therefore moved towards the person looking after him, or **pushed** so that he rolls away. The speed and direction of the 'roll' can be varied at any time.

86

Within SDM, at Key Stage 2, pupils can continue to develop body awareness and discuss the way in which their own movement ability, skills and strengths have changed/developed as they become older. At Key Stage 3, 'pupils learn about the importance of exercise', and, at Key Stage 4, 'circulation and breathing'. Both of these aspects fit very easily into SDM discussions.

Following movement experiences, where appropriate, pupils' attention can be drawn towards how they are feeling physically: 'Are you breathing heavily?'; 'Have you used a lot of energy?'; 'Do you feel tired?'; 'What happens if you have a rest?'; and following a vigorous activity, during a rest period: 'Check your pulse rate. Does it slow down after rest?'

Every movement that we make can involve the application of science, in one form or another, and, therefore, it can be argued that involvement in any form of movement can support access to National Curriculum Science. The areas in which SDM is particularly relevant are body and self-awareness within 'Forces' and 'Human Development'.

Physical Education

QCA GUIDELINES	SDM
The importance of PE to pupils with learning difficulties (p. 4) 'PE offers pupils opportunities to: • develop their skills of coordination, control, manipulation and movement'	Much of SDM's work on body awareness focuses on co-ordinated movements; for example: in a sitting position, elbows touch knees, right elbow to right knee, and then crossing right to left. Patterns are made with feet, symmetrically and asymmetrically. A lot of emphasis is put on twisting and flexibility at the waist and different ways of 'walking' using big steps/small steps, legs that are 'stiff' or legs that are 'floppy'. The 'management of body weight' is investigated through whole body movements such as rolling, jumping or somersaulting…
• develop their abilities to express themselves and be creative • …build their confidence and self-esteem.	Often these experiences are shared with a partner – *'Can you think of a way of helping your partner to jump?'* One partner can make a strong platform by kneeling on all fours, and the other partner, resting hands on their back, can then spring off the ground. Together they can work out the beginnings of 'vaulting'. Whenever appropriate, the pupils are encouraged to think of ways of working for themselves and to develop patterns of movement which are new to them. This is a fundamental aspect of Sherborne's work. Sherborne's work is not competitive – there are no winners – but that is not to say that pupils are not challenged. As a result of being encouraged to be creative and to work things out in their own way, and because any genuine effort at whatever level is celebrated and applauded, pupils are motivated to strive for progressive achievement, the attainment of which makes a very meaningful contribution towards the development of confidence and self-esteem.
Acquiring and developing skills (p. 5) 'Teaching skills development…can help pupils to: • explore, develop and establish basic movement patterns and actions they can make, *for example, the development of travelling skills that involve moving from one place to another.*'	Many of Sherborne's body awareness activities involve feeding in sensory experiences to specific parts of the body, becoming aware of those 'named' body parts moving on/over the floor and developing an awareness of how different *parts* of the body are involved and the different *ways* we can move when travelling from one place to another. Travelling **through** space considers 'pathways through space', following straight lines, curved lines, forwards/backwards, towards, away from, at all levels – floor level, in a sitting position and standing
Evaluating and improving performance (p. 6) 'Teaching this aspect…can help pupils to: • develop their listening skills and the ability to collaborate with others and share ideas when exploring different options and possibilities…and become aware of the needs of others.'	Developing an 'awareness of others' is one of the two prime objectives of Sherborne's work. Awareness of the strengths and needs of others in the group and responding sensitively is a fundamental aspect of the work. Attention is not only focused on *'me, and how I am feeling*, but also on *'what effect my actions have on other people in the group, or the person I am working with'*. It is very much a case of *'working together'*.

At each of the key stages, considerable attention is focused on 'dance' (pp. 9, 12, 15 and 19). Reading through the 'opportunities and activities' immediately suggests SDM, minus the use of music or some other external stimulus. For example, at Key Stage 1 pupils may:

> *Explore moving and/or using objects in a variety of ways in response to different types of music, for example, crawling, sliding, rolling, rocking, rowing with a partner, moving backwards, forwards and sideways...*

All of these ways of moving will be recognised as those incorporated in Sherborne's movement repertoire within body awareness, spatial activities and her relationship work, the only difference being that in SDM music is not used. Although her initial training with Rudolf Laban was in 'dance', and, in the early years, Sherborne did use music and individual musical instruments to accompany her activities, as her work evolved she came to the conclusion that she wanted us to develop the skill of 'listening to our bodies and responding accordingly' (Sherborne, 2001).

> *It is essential to help all children to concentrate on the experiences... so that they become aware of what is happening in their bodies. In this way they are able to learn from their movement experiences. I call this 'listening' to the body.* (Sherborne, 2001, p. xi)*

Music has its own character, its own rhythm, its own pitch, to which, in 'dance', we are encouraged to respond. We need opportunities to experience both 'listening to our bodies' and to 'dance'.

SDM can, however, provide an excellent basis for 'dance' in that it develops confidence in our body and its ability to move in many different ways, the confidence to move around in space in all its dimensions. It encourages creativity and allows us to explore the notion of working co-operatively with another person or group of people.

Whilst I was working in a school for children with severe learning difficulties, I was involved, with other members of staff, in a joint project between our school and a local primary school. The theme was the 'Rain Forest' and included work across the curriculum, part of which was a 'Rain Forest Dance'. In the initial stages, both groups of pupils took part in joint movement sessions, which not only served the purpose of the pupils getting to know each other through shared movement experiences, but also it gradually allowed for the exploration of particular movements which might fit into our dance. Aspects such as the size of the trees, pouring rain, very hot sun and steam, as well as a portrayal of the animals were experimented with and created in movement (See also Chapter 8).

SDM can play a very supportive roll in virtually all aspects of the PE curriculum requirements, either in a supplementary way or, in many cases, directly.

PSHE and Citizenship
A careful study of the QCA document for this subject suggests many ways in which SDM can support access in different areas. Under the heading 'Developing confidence and responsibility and making the most of their abilities' (p. 5) the document points out that:

> ...*self-concept and self-awareness:...self-esteem: the value that pupils place on themselves which is greatly influenced by the way others behave towards them...*

are of great importance. Sherborne's 'body awareness' activities, along with those concerned with 'the body in space' are aimed at, not only developing the ability to name body parts, to move about and to develop an understanding of how different parts of my body work together, but also addressing the questions, 'How do I feel about my body and its ability to move?', 'Do I have confidence in my own body's ability to move?'

As has already been pointed out in Chapter 2, one of the main aspects of Sherborne's way of working is the focus on 'success'. Providing that participation, at whatever level, is appropriate for the individual and is the result of *genuine* effort and involvement, it is celebrated and applauded. That 'celebration' is, in turn, used to motivate further effort and progress. This recognition of participation makes a very valuable contribution towards the development of a positive self-esteem:

> ...*everyone is successful in some way and everyone is praised and encouraged to pursue further effort.* (Sherborne, 2001, p. 111)*

Where appropriate, pupils are encouraged to be 'in charge' of the adults who are taking part in the session, possibly by becoming the 'supporting/caring' partner during 'with' relationship experiences, or by trying to dislodge the adult in an 'against' relationship activity. This 'changing of roles' indicates to the pupils that we *trust* them to 'look after us' or work 'against' us in the same way as we expect them to trust us when working with them. The development of a 'positive self-esteem' is one of the fundamental aspects of Sherborne's work.

The development of 'self awareness/self concept' and a positive self-esteem is a continuing theme across all of the key stages. At Key Stage 1, under the heading 'Ourselves', teachers need to ensure that *'pupils develop awareness of themselves and their bodies'* (p. 12), and this may be continued across Key Stage 2 (p. 14). At Key Stage 3, the added dimension of 'relationships' is introduced. Pupils should be given the opportunity to:

> ...*take on greater responsibility for themselves and become more aware of the views, needs and rights of others.* (p. 17)

Sherborne's 'relationship' work allows us to experience and assess how we feel about working with another person, encourages us to be aware of and sensitive towards the feelings and needs of others, and to come to decisions about how to respond, in a way which allows that shared activity to be a positive experience for both participants.

At Key Stage 4, pupils are given opportunities to:

> *...develop in confidence and independence, and take greater responsibilities in preparation for adult life.* (p. 22)

The availability of people who are able to help and give support during SDM sessions, especially when the participants are very young or need 1:1 physical support in order take part in the activities, is often a major issue when planning and implementing Sherborne's ideas. Experience has shown that, given adequate movement experience themselves at an earlier time, older students are able to offer excellent support in this way, and are very eager to do so. Not only does this allow pupils who might not be otherwise able to, to take part in sessions, but it also provides more experienced students with the opportunity to take on a very responsible role.

Participation in SDM across all the key stages gives pupils the opportunity to develop personally, in terms of how they feel about themselves, to consider how they perceive others feel about them, to develop interpersonal skills, to explore varying types of relationships in a non-judgemental and non-confrontational way, and to consider how they can work together with other people in a way which constitutes autonomy together with altruism.

There is one area, however, which, at the time of writing, is noticeably missing in any great detail from the QCA documents – that of 'the Arts'. (Happily, this is to be addressed through the setting up of a working party to look into this omission.) Carpenter and Hills write:

> *The arts in the curriculum have been sorely neglected in recent years; the lack of priority for music, dance, drama, and art within the overall National Curriculum having led to this demise.* (Carpenter and Hills, 2002, p. 22)

These writers suggest that the legacy left to us by Sherborne enables us to look at the way the Arts can make a contribution to the development of 'the whole child'. SDM, which offers participants the opportunity to develop physically, socially, emotionally and intellectually, also contains within it the opportunity to develop 'creativity' and the confidence to pursue self-expression through and alongside other art forms.

The QCA documents, which have provided one of the main references for this chapter, refer to:

> *...all pupils aged between five and 16 who have learning difficulties... this includes those who are unlikely to achieve above level 2 at Key Stage 4.*

> *(These pupils are usually described as having severe or profound and multiple learning difficulties.)*

This was the group of children with whom Sherborne originally developed her work. However, over the years, it has become apparent that the use of SDM can be very beneficial across the whole spectrum of special needs. Moreover, bearing in mind the full title of her book, *Developmental Movement for Children: Mainstream, special needs and pre-school*, where it has been used with pupils in the mainstream setting it has been very successful, especially in the area of social skills and social awareness through relationship movement experiences. It is an ideal vehicle for the development of interpersonal skills at all levels of ability.

Inclusion

Extensive discussion and debate centres, at the present time, on the subject of 'inclusion'. It is a complex subject presenting what could be regarded as the greatest challenge to educators at the present time. To date, encompassing all aspects which typify everyday society, Florian et al. (1998) suggest that 'a truly satisfactory definition has yet to emerge', but in terms of education, 'inclusion' is based on the belief in:

> *... the right of all children with special educational needs to the same educational opportunity as that available to other children.* (Florian et al., 1998, p. 2)

At the same time, they recognise that:

> *...it is the acceptance of difference that is the hallmark of inclusive practice.* (Ibid., p. 23)

In his very challenging and thought-provoking chapter, 'The curriculum – a vehicle for inclusion or a lever for exclusion', Rose suggests that:

> *... of all the areas of change which are required for the promotion of inclusion, it is that of attitude which will provide the greater obstacle.* (Rose, 1996, p. 28)

'Inclusion', if it is genuinely to become what it says, both philosophically and in terms of implementation, must be undertaken with an absolute belief in, and commitment to, the principles involved within it. It will take, on the part of many teachers both in mainstream and existing special needs provision, a complete review of teaching styles, methods of curriculum delivery and attitude towards the rights and value of pupils with special educational needs. As Gerschel (1998) writes, 'The concept of equal value is essential to inclusive education'. Furthermore, applying this to classroom activities:

> *... consideration should... be given to creating favourable classroom conditions where pupils learn to value working together,* (Marven, 1998, p. 146)

whilst bearing in mind that:

> *... the concept of total inclusion is of course a goal, an aim towards which all endeavours are directed.* (Tilstone, 1998, p. 160)

There will always be some pupils whose needs are such – maybe in terms of multiple sensory impairments, profound and multiple learning difficulties or extreme challenging behaviour – that they will need some form of special provision. As Steele (1998) notes, 'It is important to remember that inclusion is a process that occurs over time' and that that process will take a great deal of innovative thinking before its objectives are fully met.

In the second edition of the highly acclaimed book, *Enabling Access* (2001), the editors, Barry Carpenter, Rob Ashdown and Keith Bovair write, in the introductory chapter:

> *Central to this debate [on inclusion] should be the rights of the child as a learner. How do we design learning environments and learning activities that will ensure that each child is an active participant in the learning process and not a bystander, a peripheral participant, watching the activities of others?* (Carpenter et al., 2001, p. 2)

Referring back to how QCA Guidelines can be cross-referenced with some of Sherborne's movement experiences and philosophy, I would put forward SDM as one of the key providers of such an activity. In SDM activities, pupils of *all* abilities are able to work together, and everyone's contribution is equally valued and celebrated within a shared learning environment, while their 'differences' are recognised.

A significant part of this chapter has been assigned to showing how SDM can support access to the National Curriculum in the core subjects of English, Mathematics and Science and also in PE and PSHE and Citizenship. However, the use of SDM in education is not confined to pupils in the pre-school–16 years age range. It also offers an ideal opportunity for some post-16 students to take on the role of carers/helpers in groups where additional supporters would be an advantage or, indeed, necessary. Given that these students will have previously experienced SDM for themselves, they take on this supporting role very diligently, and respond very ably and positively to the responsibility encapsulated within it.

Finally, within the present education system, SDM comes 'full circle', in that there are examples of it being used very successfully in varying contexts with students in higher education.

The Use of SDM in Higher Education

Remembering that Sherborne first used her movement ideas with students who were attending Initial Teacher Training courses in Bristol, it is interesting to note how SDM is still being used in higher education. As my own experience has been predominantly within the pre-school to 19-year age range, I have relied on the experience and expertise of my Sherborne Association colleagues to cover this important application of Sherborne's ideas. George Hill, Dr Elizabeth Marsden, Bill Richards and Janet Sparkes have provided the following pieces, which outline their use of SDM at various higher education establishments in the UK.

❖

George Hill, working with the University of Bristol

The tutor responsible for the Social Work course at Bristol University approached me about running an SDM session for his students. This was for activities of choice during the last week of the course before graduation. I was able to provide a 2-hour session, which was greatly approved by the participants. It gave them the opportunity to relax and **'play'** *together in a non-challenging way. The post-course evaluation showed the SDM session as the most popular; the students commented that it gave them the opportunity of making good, positive relationships with their fellow students without the fear of any embarrassment. These improved relationships were noted with interest by the tutor.*

Following discussions with the tutor, we decided that running an SDM session at the beginning of the next course might well be a way of rapidly establishing a good group identity – hopefully replacing a gradual build up to such an identity. At the start of the next course, we ran an SDM session on the second day. This session was run with particular thought given to the needs and feelings of the mature students. It was necessary to allow the students to become relaxed and comfortable within their own bodies and feelings. Therefore the first experiences were for the individual building up of self-understanding and self-confidence – well in line with Sherborne's theories of knowledge of self, followed by knowledge of others. Having built up good self-images, we then started to go through experiences which built up knowledge of others, leading to trust and good positive relationships. This was a success; it was pleasing to see the change taking place in the students. The session had started with some embarrassment and giggling. This had now changed to very relaxed laughing and a growing understanding of each other's strengths and areas of need. A very good group relationship had been achieved – a 'relationship' which proved very important in the subsequent group activities which formed part of the course. Again, the end-of-course evaluations proved the point. SDM was declared one of the best inputs with a request that a session might also be arranged at the end of each course. This was agreed by the tutor who said that the SDM had made particular aspects of the course very successful compared with previous years. SDM became a regular feature of those particular courses.

Dr Elizabeth Marsden, University of Paisley (Ayr Campus)
*At Aberdeen University, the Counselling Department tried to assist students with exam phobia and generalised fears (e.g. being away from home, financial problems, lack of coping ability, depression). They held sessions by psychologists, and I ran one based on SDM with a marked emphasis on (1) being at home with themselves, and (2) using physical means of relating to others. These SDM sessions were related as being **the** most beneficial sessions. I did not do any research with these groups, but my perception was that having time out to focus on, accept and come to terms with one's own physical presence was as important to these fearful students as was learning to relate to others.*

*With primary education students, I continue to use SDM for two main purposes. Firstly, when sensitively taught, it is a very non-threatening introduction to PE. Most of the primary education students have not enjoyed PE at school, and yet they know they must learn how to teach it to primary children, so they dread their PE input. By introducing SDM, it gives the students some security because they are not competing in games (most of them think this is what PE is all about); they are having time out to reconnect to their physical self without having to compare themselves with others (i.e. they can **all** feel successful and, once connected to their physical self, they can feel a sense of security and mastery which leads to self-confidence). They may also feel less threatened by SDM, as initially there may be a lot of movement at floor level rather than from standing. Operating at standing level can also make some feel vulnerable and more visible to others.*

Secondly, primary students who are just starting their education course may not know each other or the PE tutor. This adds to their feelings of anxiety in PE, since they do not have the security of hiding behind desks in a classroom. Being in a wide space such as a gym or hall can make people feel very noticeable and visible. Starting a course with SDM will give students the chance to get to know their class-mates and the tutor in a completely different way from the normal social mechanisms. SDM is an icebreaker and a barrier blower. Relating to someone by pushing, pulling or sliding their body weight is totally different to trying to strike up a conversation. Being slid around by one's feet negates any attempt at looking cool in the eyes of the slider!

Students who have already worked together as a class (maybe Year 2 or 3 students) will be amazed how they will see each other in a completely new way after using SDM. This is especially obvious during care giving and care receiving when one participant is blindfolded. Once the blindfold is removed that 'blinded' student is always incredulous that such-and-such was their partner. Because the sense of sight is so important in the relationships we build up with each other, the sense of touch is rarely used. In SDM, it is always used, and it brings into play a completely new understanding of others.

*SDM is based on the philosophy of Laban, but is not defined by it, and its use with primary student teachers helps their understanding of how to **apply** Laban. It also challenges the preconceptions that most students have about PE (that it is* *'games') and helps them to focus on **movement** education. SDM is also a great example of how good movement teaching can accommodate the principles of inclusion.*

Bill Richards, with John Dibbo and Maureen Douglas, Senior Lecturers, Rolle College of Education, University of Plymouth

On taking up a new post as a lecturer in PE at Rolle College of Higher Education with the responsibility of preparing students for the teaching of the PE curriculum in primary schools, I had to develop a starting point – and quickly! I had taken on the position half-way through an academic year, I was the only lecturer in the 'team', and I did not inherit any course structure!

I started with a four-week course in SDM for all the student groups. I recognised that the students would bring a range of experiences to these sessions, some seeming positive, but many anxious at the thought of PE. They told me afterwards that it was unlike any PE that they had been involved in, and that it was fun. It helped them to relax with their own bodies, and begin to develop the understanding and confidence to approach the more traditional areas of the physical curriculum (e.g. Gymnastics).

This starting point was very significant for the future direction and development of PE at Rolle, which became a Polytechnic and eventually the Rolle School of Education in the University of Plymouth. During this time, the full team increased to three lecturers with additional part-time support. Together, we developed a course in PE for students opting to specialise in the primary sector. The basis of the course was constructed on the following three aims:

- *An understanding of the whole child through the study of developmental patterns*
- *An understanding of the theory and practice developed by Rudolf Laban, and*
- *An understanding of the theory and practice of SDM.*

This provided the conceptual framework from which the students explored the physical curriculum. It was a unique course, developed through the experience and beliefs of the team and positively explored by the students. We believed, as a team, that in order for students to develop into effective and inspiring teachers, they needed to understand their own bodies and movement potential. SDM provided one of the significant means of reaching this aim.

Janet Sparkes, Principal Lecturer, Head of Schools Partnerships, King Alfred's College of Higher Education, Winchester

This statement on the use of SDM in higher education has a particular focus on students following an Initial Teacher Training course in Primary Education. Although, over a period of many years, students training to work with children and adults with physical and learning difficulties have covered courses in SDM in some depth, other students following a degree course in Primary Education have been recipients of SDM as part of their curriculum development in

Movement/PE. Some of these students would have been following a specialist pathway in PE as part of their Primary Education route, whilst the majority would have been non-specialist movement students. The focus of this piece is on the latter two groups of students with whom, initially, SDM has been used specifically to build a positive attitude to the experience of movement.

Meeting higher education students for the first time in a movement context can be a challenge for the teacher and those taught. It is important to be aware of feelings and perceptions of students in that particular environment. For some, memories and, therefore, present perceptions are negative because of experiences of failure in PE; for others, there is a personal level of competence as a participant in sports and movement activities which can be a barrier to analysing the stages that have contributed to movement confidence and competence.

Over the years, adopting a SDM approach to students' initial movement/PE classes has proved invaluable. Sessions have been structured with the goals of breaking down 'movement prejudices', of creating a non-threatening learning context where the experiences are positive, fun, enhancing and individual, and contribute to group comfortableness. There are no named skills to master (or not), but engagement with the body that allows every individual to work at a personal level, free from comparison and the possible humiliation of failure. The challenge can be set in such a way that the less competent and the more competent can find a level of working that satisfies a personal need and ability. An initial emphasis on working individually and, therefore, finding a personal level of working can move gradually to engaging with a partner where the emphasis is on finding ways to co-operate – a less threatening behavioural response for the less competent mover. Testing your partner in 'battles' of strength does not always conform to the expected norms, and more often than not results in unconstrained laughter! Developing movement sensitivity, movement awareness and basic movement abilities happens naturally.

As a teacher, I am also aware that the movement experience in which I am engaging the students can be analysed and discussed retrospectively, not only in terms of the social and emotional concepts identified above, but also in relation to some of the language and concepts that the students will need to understand and apply as potential teachers of PE to primary age children; for example, developing body awareness, sensing changes of quality in movement, thinking about the space the mover occupies, noting the influence of others whilst moving.

Where did I start? Using the ideas shared in this book with the purpose of students having fun. Initially, there is little pre-explanation; there is more commentary as the students work on bodily demands, the kinaesthetic feelings, the different partnerships and groupings that are experienced. The movement language is used naturally in the setting with limited focus in the early stage on more in-depth analysis.

On this foundation, the movement can be fun and can engage the individual in different social contexts. Trust and openness can be built. Students are encouraged to share feelings and perceptions in a non-technical way and using non-technical language initially. A dialogue can begin which can move very naturally to the language the student needs to engage with as they learn to analyse movement, to deconstruct and construct certain movement experiences. SDM can introduce the student to a wide range of movement skills, movement knowledge and understanding that are at the heart of a sound PE curriculum. Not only have I found this approach to the early stages of students' movement training beneficial in making sense of that important fundamental movement phase of motor development, but also I have found myself returning to the principles and practices of SDM as the students progress in their understanding of a PE programme.

❖

Following these accounts of the use of SDM in higher education, and having touched briefly on the subject of 'inclusion', and incorporated information on the use of SDM in Initial Teacher Training, I would suggest that SDM can undoubtedly make a very valuable and significant contribution both for future teachers and pupils in many areas of education. Firstly, it is a very meaningful way of allowing pupils to work together. It is a way in which *everyone's* contribution and participation can be equally valued and celebrated, and which fosters confidence in self and a respect and consideration for others. Secondly, in terms of Initial Teacher Training, an understanding of the basic theory and philosophy which underpins Sherborne's work would make a valuable contribution towards the development of the ethos necessary to influence the attitudes required if 'inclusion' is to be meaningfully implemented in the future.

This chapter has covered a broad spectrum of the beneficial use of SDM in education, encompassing work with pupils and students with learning difficulties, its application within the field of higher education in terms of Initial Teacher Training, and as an 'ice-breaker' for students on other higher education courses. SDM offers access to the basic teaching and learning processes and experiences right across the curriculum, not only to pupils with special needs, but also, in some areas, to pupils in the mainstream setting and higher education.

References
Carpenter, B., Ashdown, R. and Bovair, K. (eds) (2001) *Enabling Access: Effective teaching and learning for pupils with learning difficulties* (2nd edn). London: David Fulton.
Carpenter, B. and Hills P. (2002) 'Rescuing the Arts', *SLD Experience*, Spring edition.
Florian, L., Rose, R. and Tilstone, C. (eds) (1998) *Promoting Inclusive Practice*. London: Routledge.
Gershel, L. (1998) 'Equal opportunities and special educational needs: equity and inclusion'. In: L. Florian, R. Rose and C. Tilstone (eds) *Promoting Inclusive Practice*. London: Routledge.

Marven, C. (1998) 'Individual and whole class teaching'. In: L. Florian, R. Rose and C. Tilstone (eds) *Promoting Inclusive Practice.* London: Routledge.

Qualifications and Curriculum Authority (QCA) (2001) *Guidelines for Planning, Teaching and Assessing the Curriculum for Pupils with Special Needs* [English, Mathematics, Science, Physical Education and Personal, Social and Health Education and Citizenship]. London: QCA.

Rose, R. (1998) 'The curriculum: a vehicle for inclusion or a lever for exclusion'. In: L. Florian, R. Rose and C. Tilstone (eds) *Promoting Inclusive Practice.* London: Routledge.

Sherborne, V. (2001) *Developmental Movement for Children: Mainstream, special needs and pre-school* (2nd edn). London: Worth Publishing.

Steele, J. (1998) 'Routes to inclusion'. In: L. Florian, R. Rose and C. Tilstone (eds) *Promoting Inclusive Practice.* London: Routledge.

Tilstone, C. (1998) 'Moving towards reality'. In: L. Florian, R. Rose and C. Tilstone (eds) *Promoting Inclusive Practice.* London: Routledge.

*Reprinted by kind permission of Worth Publishing from *Developmental Movement for Children* by Veronica Sherborne.
2nd Edition. Worth Publishing Limited 2001.

PART 3

Questions, Suggestions and Projects

CHAPTER 7
Some Frequently Asked Questions, with Answers and Suggestions

Q1. Can I use music with Sherborne Developmental Movement (SDM)?

A1. This is perhaps the question most frequently asked by SDM course participants. The answer lies within the distinction between (a) 'doing SDM' and (b) 'using Sherborne's ideas' in varying contexts.

a) If we are doing SDM, then we *do not* use music. In her early films with students, *In Touch* and *Explorations*, we see Sherborne using musical instruments, music and her voice to accompany her movement experiences. As her work with children began to develop, she came to the conclusion that she wanted participants to 'listen to their bodies'. In the introduction to her book, she writes:

> *…it is essential to help children to concentrate on the experiences…so that they become aware of what is happening to their bodies. I call this 'listening to the body'.* (Sherborne, 2001, p. xiv)*

Music has its own rhythms and qualities which could be distracting in this respect.

b) However, in the summary of her book she says:

> *Each teacher can make use of the material described in this book in his or her own way. Teachers develop their own variations and ideas, as do the children they teach.* (Ibid., p. 111)*

She points out that her work can provide a foundation for gymnastics, sports and dance, and as a preparation for drama. If we are 'using Sherborne's ideas' in another context, and music is appropriate, then there is no reason why we should not use it to accompany the activity. Indeed, it can be argued that music can offer a release to some of us who may be otherwise reluctant to 'move' for whatever reason.

It is a matter of being clear in our minds about the difference between 'doing SDM' as outlined in Sherborne's book, and 'using Sherborne's ideas' in varying contexts.

Q2. What do I do if I have someone in the group who does not want to join in?

A2. Providing that person is not disrupting the group, try not to react to him. The chances are that, when he sees other participants enjoying themselves and becoming involved, he will want to join in and come back of his own accord. If he persists in disruptive behaviour, I would first involve him in a

1:1 relationship with a supporter. If this did not work, and he continued to disrupt the work of the rest of the group, I would remove him from the group and have him sit out on the side, under supervision if necessary, allowing him to return to the group if this became appropriate. It is very rare, apart from some instances when working with participants who are on the autistic spectrum, that 'reluctant participants' do not eventually return to the group of their own accord.

Q3. How do I respond if someone appears not to like a particular activity?

A3. Keep trying; do not give up immediately. Often someone who is sensitively encouraged to participate, even though this may involve a degree of physical intervention, will find it enjoyable once he is experiencing the activity, and in time will relax and take part. If you do have someone in the group who is particularly sensitive, it is sometimes helpful for that person to work with a regular partner to build up a stable relationship until confidence is established. Of course, if the negative response to a particular activity persists for some reason, then it would be wrong to continue to pursue it with that person. It would be better at that time to offer an experience which he is known to enjoy, and then come back to the previous experience perhaps next time. One of the important aspects of SDM is 'flexibility' (see Chapter 2) If a particular approach does not produce a positive outcome for any reason, be prepared to try something else.

Q4. How would you sum up the main benefits of using SDM?

A4. SDM, used on a regular basis, makes a very positive contribution towards the personal development of the participants in terms of:

- The development of trust and confidence in self and others, resulting in a very positive working relationship between group leaders, supporters and participants, thus enhancing the teaching/learning environment
- The development of interpersonal skills, a sensitivity towards the feelings of others and a sense of altruism
- Successful participation in physical activities at whatever skill level is appropriate for the individual
- An opportunity to explore the concept of how individuals feel about themselves and others, and how they perceive others think of them
- An opportunity to experience 'success' and 'creativity', leading to the development of a positive self-image and self-esteem
- An opportunity to take part in physical activity in which all participants can achieve a successful outcome, thus contributing towards health and well-being.

(See Chapters 2 and 3; and 'Developmental Movement – a summary' (p. 111) in Sherborne, 2001.)

Q5. What would you say were the main issues surrounding the use of SDM?

A5. The main issues concerned with the practical implementation of SDM are:

- The issue of 'touch' must be clarified, and if necessary resolved, before any movement sessions can take place. Check on organisational policies which are in place, and, if necessary, gain permission from parents or carers before starting movement sessions. It is sometimes helpful to explain to them the nature and benefits of the work before you begin.
- Physical implications of activities for the student need also to be assessed before you begin SDM sessions, especially when working with participants who have profound and multiple learning difficulties. In this case, it is best to check with the physiotherapist beforehand that none of the experiences you have planned are contra-indicated for the individuals concerned.
- 'Lifting' is a big issue, as your and the supporters' physical well-being is as important as that of the participants, especially if you are working with people who are non-ambulant. The necessary use of hoists and other appliances brings in the additional issues of 'time', and the number of helpers and supporters you are able to call on. You have to be realistic, and bear in mind the safety of all concerned. Blankets and duvet covers – one for each participant to lie or sit on – cuts down waiting time between activities.
- There are many general issues surrounding the use of SDM – e.g. why it cannot be done with particular groups of people – but invariably these 'problems', when approached with an open mind and positive attitude, can be resolved to a degree, if not entirely. Keeping the work simple and floor-based will go a long way towards solving these issues in many instances.

(See Chapter 4.)

Q6. Is it possible to do SDM with participants who are on the autistic spectrum and who may be tactile defensive?

A6. Work with participants on the autistic spectrum needs special consideration:

- Contrary to the basic principles of SDM, it is sometimes helpful to have a set routine, especially for the beginning and ending of the session. An arrangement of mats can help to form a 'focus' for the group.
- Use blankets for sliding, hoops as a 'link' contact, large 'scrunch rings' as a physical medium for linking the group.
- Physical contact can sometimes be made through the back, so there is no eye-contact. Small participants may lie on the back of a supporter and be taken for a slide.
- Work with 1:1 support (2:1 at the most). Your supporters should have a good awareness of SDM, as you should be prepared to have varying activities going on at the same time, according to the needs and preferences of the individuals in the group. If this happens, it is important to ensure that everyone comes together at intervals during the session and at the end.

(See Chapters 2 and 4.)

Q7. How do I begin and end my sessions, and how would you suggest I organise my first SDM sessions?

A7. How you begin your first SDM session will depend on the nature of your group, but, as a general rule, begin and end with everyone – participants, supporters and yourself – sitting on the floor together. If you are working with younger, partnered participants or those who require 1:1 support, then begin with the partners sitting together, either next to each other or with the supporting partner sitting behind the younger or less able participant. If you are working with older participants, it is more appropriate, and very likely, that they will prefer to sit in their own space. With younger children, Sherborne suggested we begin with 'relationship experiences' to build up the trust and confidence between participant and carer (see Part 1 in Sherborne, 2001), but, with older participants and groups of physically able children, individual activities (sliding on hips or stomachs; greeting those you meet) may be deemed more appropriate.

- At the beginning of your first movement session, explain that: 'We are all going to be doing something new – and at the end of the session we will talk about how we felt about it.' Start with very simple movement experiences (e.g. sliding either alone or with partner as appropriate). Develop this by trying 'spinning on hips' and 'sliding in different directions, at different speeds'. In the early stages, change the movement fairly frequently in order to avoid boredom with an activity. At a later stage, when your participants have had more movement experience, you will be able to allow more time for individual exploration and creativity.
- Vary the movement qualities (see Chapter 1) in terms of: spatial dimensions – forwards, backwards, side to side, spinning around; time – fast and slow; weight – strong and gentle movements; and bound and stiff and free flow movements to sustain interest.
- In follow-up sessions, summarise and build on previous sessions.
- If *you* are new to the work, have a list of the 'experiences' you intend to offer – maybe on the back of your hand! – just in case you forget what you intended to do. You will be able to dispense with the list as your confidence grows. With experience, you will be able to take a more flexible approach, taking ideas from the group.
- Remember to include experiences which include some body awareness, some work on space, some relationship experiences and opportunities for 'creativity'.
- Work on 'contrasts': if you have been doing something which has been very energetic, follow this with a calm, gentle movement; follow something fast with a slow movement, etc.
- As at the beginning, end the session with participants together as a group in a quiet and calming atmosphere. It is important that sessions end in a relaxed but structured way.

I would suggest that your early movement sessions last no longer than 20 minutes, allowing time at the beginning and at the end for taking off and putting on shoes and socks. In terms of managing the group dynamics, it is helpful to keep the participants 'grounded/floor-based' in your early sessions.

(See Chapter 4.)

Q8. What should I do if the participants I am working with find it difficult to sit still on the floor or in a structured group?

A8. This could well be the case if you are working with participants who have (a) attention deficit/hyperactivity disorder or (b) are on the autistic spectrum. In both cases, you need a 1:1 ratio (or at the most 2:1) of support. In the case of group (a):

- These people are almost perpetually in free flow/fast mode in terms of their movements, and this is where we must begin with them: running – stopping – jumping – touch them as they run past – catch them – swing them (if they are small enough) – let them go again – gradually build in a structure which is challenging for them but at the same time fun!
- The structure needs to be very simple to start with: running – stopping – changing direction – running – sitting down – running again. All very energetic!
- Gradually 'ground' them until they will sit for a short period of time before moving again, and, if they are ready for it, maybe walking this time.
- Once the group is 'grounded', try giving individual slides or rolling – keeping the energy levels high, but gradually introducing slower movements: sliding on backs, stomachs – fast and then 'very slowly' to emphasise the contrast.
- Be prepared to run sessions on these lines over a period of at least five or six sessions – it may take more – gradually introducing more structure and partner work.
- Try to end each session with everyone together as a group, either sitting by their partner, or, if possible, being quietly 'cradled' – but, if this is the case, do not hold this too long in the early stages.

In the case of group (b), refer to Q6.

Q9. Can I do SDM if I have not got access to a 'slidey' floor

A9. This does make your sessions more difficult to run, as so many of Sherborne's movement experiences are based on 'sliding', but it is possible to overcome this difficulty to a certain extent:

- It is possible to cover a designated area with mats, providing they are all of the same thickness. The ones with 'Velcro' attaching sides are most successful, as un-joined mats tend to move apart when people are sliding over them.
- Heavy plastic is a possibility, but this can become sticky and uncomfortable in hot weather, and *must* be secured at the edges for reasons of safety.
- Perhaps the best solution is the use of medium to large picnic type rugs/mats, used plastic side down; these will slide over a carpeted area and can be used for partner work.

Q10. Is it possible to work with mixed ability groups?
A10. This is an ideal situation, which encompasses Sherborne's philosophy that all those who participate in her movement experiences are able to succeed at their own level and are equally valued:

- More able participants can help and support participants who may have physical difficulties.
- More experienced participants can help and support newcomers to SDM.
- Older participants can support younger ones.
- Mainstream pupils can work alongside pupils with special needs, on an equal basis or in a supporting role.
- Less able participants can model their movements on those of the more able ones.

It is important that *anyone* who is taking on a helping/supporting role has the opportunity of becoming aware of the basic principles and practical aspects of SDM beforehand. Ideally, this should be in the form of taking part in introductory sessions or at least having the opportunity of watching video examples of the work.

In general terms, there is absolutely no claim that SDM is suitable for everyone, and, for individuals who do not feel comfortable with the work, there must be an acceptance of this and respect for their feelings. For some participants, the aspect of physical contact and touch may be too much to overcome. For some would-be session leaders, the necessary teaching styles may not be compatible with how they view their role – all these aspects must be respected and acknowledged.

There is certainly no claim that SDM has all the answers, but, in most cases, given time and a supportive environment, there are very few situations where participation in an SDM session results in a totally negative experience for the vast majority of those taking part. Alongside many other methods of working, especially with individuals with disability or need, it should be viewed as an additional, very useful and beneficial 'tool' for anyone who is involved in any way in work with people and their personal development.

References

Sherborne, V. (2001) *Developmental Movement for Children: Mainstream, special needs and pre-school* (2nd edn). London: Worth Publishing.

*Reprinted by kind permission of Worth Publishing from *Developmental Movement for Children* by Veronica Sherborne. 2nd Edition. Worth Publishing Limited 2001.

CHAPTER 8
The Sherborne Developmental Movement/Science Project

During the Spring Term 2002, as part of a 'Science Week', I was invited to lead workshops on 'sound and light' for lower school pupils with severe and multiple learning difficulties at Warmley Park School, on the outskirts of Bristol. My remit was to include some of the properties of light and sound, and to reflect those properties in movement and dance.

I decided to work on two basic themes:

- Light travels in 'straight' lines
- Sound can travel in 'curved' lines and can go around corners.

I linked the science and Sherborne Developmental Movement (SDM) in the following way:

SCIENCE THEMES	SDM THEMES
Light *Properties of light:* • Illuminating • Travels in straight lines • Cannot go around corners	*Characterised by:* 'Direct' pathways through space – moving in straight or zigzag lines, marching movements, straight arms swinging in all directions
Sound *Properties of sound:* • Cannot see it • Can travel around corners • Can be heard even though source is not visible	*Characterised by:* 'Flexible' pathways through space – sliding on stomachs, rolling

(See also 'Laban's Movement Analysis', Chapter 1.)

The pupils were divided into four groups: (1) Reception; (2) Years 1 and 2; (3) Years 3 and 4; and (4) Years 5 and 6. A further group was made up of the pupils from the units for pupils on the autistic spectrum. It was decided that those pupils who made up the latter group should work separately, allowing me the option of running an alternative workshop for them based on movement experiences already familiar to them should they not respond to the contents of the dance workshop. All the pupils were asked to bring in a torch, and the workshops took place in the school hall, which had been darkened and then illuminated, using revolving light patterns. Prior to the workshops, I had selected three pieces of music: one which suggested quick, 'sparky' movements for 'light', a piece which was much slower and lower in tone to accompany 'sound', and finally a bright joyful piece for the culmination of 'the dance'.

I have allowed my session plan, reproduced below, to describe the session.

Organisation and workshop plan
Duration of each workshop – 1 hour

Equipment
Large torch for personal use
A large box, covered in silver hologram paper (open on one side, to act as a screen)
A selection of musical instruments which reflected the properties of light and sound (high pitched for light – low pitched for sound)
Coloured streamers
Stereo tape deck

Ask all pupils to bring in a torch.

Introduction to the Workshop
1. Invite pupils and helpers to come and sit on the floor in front of the box (containing a large torch and selected instruments).
2. Greet each pupil, 'finding' them with the torch beam.
3. Shine the torch around the hall – get pupils to 'track' it.
4. Ask pupils to listen to the sounds made by each of the instruments.
5. Ask questions, such as 'Do they sound the same?'; 'How are the sounds "different"?'

Development of the Science Theme
1. Shine the torch towards pupils – 'Can you see the light?' – Yes!
2. Hide the torch in the box – 'Can you see the light?' – No!
3. Shine the torch towards pupils – 'Can you see the light now?' – Yes!
4. Repeat 2.
5. Explanation: light can travel only in straight lines; it cannot turn corners to 'get out of the box'.
6. Play the musical instruments in view of pupils – 'Can you see the instruments?' – Yes!; 'Can you hear the sound?' – Yes!
7. Play the instruments in the box – 'Can you see the instruments'? – No!; 'Can you hear the sound?' – Yes!
8. Explanation: Even when you cannot see the instruments, you can still hear the sound. That is because sound can travel in curved lines and can go around corners to get out of the box and reach your ears.

Development of the Movement/Dance Theme
1. Practise 'light movements': 'direct' pathways through space – marching – changing direction – zigzag movements.
2. Practise 'sound movements': 'flexible' pathways through space – sliding on stomachs – rolling.

3. Repeat 1 and 2 using appropriate musical instruments.
4. Repeat introducing selected music, using torches with 'light dance' movements, and streamers with 'sound dance' music.

The Dance
1. Divide pupils and helpers into 'sound dancers' and 'light dancers', and seat them in a circle.
2. 'Sound dancers', with streamers, wait in a group away from 'light dancers'.
3. 'Light dance' – to the sound of the 'light dance' music:
   a) 'Light dancers' form a square and move around the square, using marching movements and 'dancing' with torches
   b) Dancers turn and dance in other direction
   c) Dancers move into the middle of the square and out again
   d) Repeat (a).
4. On hearing 'sound dance' music, 'light dancers' go into centre of circle and 'huddle' in a 'frightened' group.
5. 'Sound dancers' roll or slide towards light dancers – wave streamers – touch them with streamers.
6. 'Light dancers' are no longer 'frightened', and join the 'sound dancers'.
7. Free dance: 'light dancers' and 'sound dancers' join together and dance together to the third piece of selected music. When it begins to fade, all come to the centre and sit together, waving streamers and torches. Gradually fade music and movements.

Conclusion to the workshop
1. Review the properties of sound and light.
2. Discuss how those properties were represented in 'the dance'.
3. Ask pupils to express their feelings about their experience.

Summary
All groups appeared to enjoy taking part in the workshops. Non-ambulant pupils were either carried, if they were small, or participated in their wheelchairs. It was delightful to see some of the smallest pupils making their way into the hall at the beginning of their workshop almost weighed down by enormous torches, which seemed almost as big as themselves, hanging around their necks! I was particularly pleased with the response of the group made up of pupils on the autistic spectrum. With 1:1, or at the least 1:2 support, they took full part in all the practical aspects of their workshop, and certainly enjoyed 'the dance'.

The workshops proved to be a very good example of the successful way in which SDM can support access to the National Curriculum, whilst at the same time offering participants an enjoyable and creative experience.

Since our 'dance/science' experience, I have had the opportunity to read Peppy Hills' very inspiring book, *It's Your Move*, and I was very interested to learn how closely her underpinning philosophy regarding the implementation of her work matched that of SDM. She speaks of a crucial starting point as working 'with the dancers as they are – here and now' (Hills, 2003) and the importance of the relationship between the dancer and the support worker, who 'may need to give input at times…sensitively and without taking over.' (Ibid.). Throughout the book, there are many examples of ways of working, which are also applied to SDM. This, for me, is a very positive and strengthening observation in that it substantiates and fortifies both SDM and 'the dance', and underpins the collective qualities of the experiences being offered, in both cases, to the participants.

References
Hills. P. (2003) *It's Your Move*. Birmingham: Questions Publishing Company.

CHAPTER 9
Research Projects
Recent and On-going

The Action Research Project

Although the teaching styles and approach adopted in the implementation of Sherborne Developmental Movement (SDM) are very subjective, the use of Sherborne's ideas must stand up to the test of objective scrutiny and research. As I have already said in the introduction, it is not enough simply to say, 'It works!' We must ask ourselves why it works, and also whether or not these subjective claims can be substantiated? As pointed out by Hopkins:

> *The challenge is to capitalise on the current demands for accountability by emphasising professionalism rather than some arbitrary output criteria.*
> (Hopkins, 1985, p. 120)

Having used Sherborne's ideas with my particular class group over a considerable period of time, I became convinced that the movement did have a noticeable effect on the classroom behaviour of the pupils. I therefore decided to set up a research project which would test my thinking and observations objectively. I subsequently ran a research project similar to the one described in this chapter for which the results were very encouraging. However, it could be argued that those pupils had already had considerable movement experience and that this could have influenced the results. For this reason, I decided to repeat the project again recently, but this time with another teacher working with a group of children who had had very little previous exposure to Sherborne's ideas.

One of the claims made by Sherborne is that:

> *If children learn to use their strength in a focused way... they will develop skills in attending.* (Sherborne, 2001, p. 31)*

Accepting that:

> *...perceptual development in childhood is largely a matter of the development of attention,* (Shaffer, 1996, p. 228)

and that:

> *...as children's attention spans increase, they are better able to plan what they will attend to and to ignore distractions,* (Ibid., p. 307)

I decided to take as the first part of my hypothesis that:

SDM can contribute towards an increase in the ability to attend and stay 'on task'.

In the summary at the end of her book, under the heading of 'Development of personality', Sherborne claims that:

> *They [the children] learn to become sensitive to the needs and feelings of others and become more skilled in communicating and sharing experiences with other people.* (Sherborne, 2001, p. 111)*

On the subject of altruism (see Chapter 3) – the ability to feel and show concern for others – Shaffer suggests that one way of developing this is by:

> *...structuring play activities so that children are likely to discover the benefits of co-operating and helping one another.* (Shaffer, 1996, p. 566)

As discussed in Chapter 2, the development of an 'awareness of others' is one of the two prime objectives of Sherborne's work. Intrinsic within all of her 'relationship' work is the development of a growing awareness of the person/people you are working with: 'How are they feeling?'; 'Do they have the necessary trust and confidence in me to view our shared experiences in a positive way?'; 'Am I making them feel threatened in any way?'; 'Do I have an understanding of what this feels like for them?'; 'Can we work together in a positive way, taking into account how each of us are feeling?' With these aspects of 'awareness of others' and 'social interaction' in mind, I decided to set as the second part of my hypothesis the premise that:

SDM can enhance the development of positive social interaction.

I wanted the research to be undertaken in the normal classroom setting, using situations which fell naturally into the timetable and classroom routines, with the absolute minimum of change or disruption. This led me to adopt what Shaffer (1996) describes as the 'correlation design' of research, in which:

> *... the investigator gathers information to determine whether two or more variables of interest are meaningfully related... no attempts are made to manipulate the participants' environment in any way.* (Ibid., p. 20)

The 'variables' which formed the basis of this investigation were simply 'non-movement' and 'movement'. The method of data collection consisted of **observing and recording** behaviour in the classroom, then repeating the process, making *exactly* the same observations, but, this time, immediately following a movement session, and comparing the two results.

As I was interested in the effect that SDM would have on the everyday classroom behaviour of the children, I felt it was important that there was as little disruption to the classroom routine as possible. I appreciated from the outset that such conditions would carry the possibility of the influence of external incidents, which could influence behaviour and consequently the data obtained, and so decided to work under the umbrella of 'action research':

A feature which makes action research a very suitable procedure for work in classrooms and schools is its flexibility and adaptability... These qualities are revealed in the changes that may take place during its implementation and in the course of on-the-spot experimentation and innovation characterizing the approach... Action research relies chiefly on observation and behavioural data. (Cohen and Marion, 1984, p. 47)

Hopkins (1985) suggests that there are two approaches to classroom action research – closed and open. In the former, the hypothesis has already been identified and is subsequently tested; the latter, 'open' approach is a more reflective activity in that there is an emergence of a hypothesis/idea which can then be tested. This project fell into the 'closed' approach category in that I had been using SDM over a period of several years, had observed what I felt were the benefits to the class group, and consequently decided to scrutinise those beliefs using a form of research methodology.

Setting Up the Method of Data Collection

I decided to use the same research instruments that I had used previously. These were based on the principles of the Flanders Interaction Analysis Categories (FIAC). The format for the observation schedules was developed from those used by Croll (1986), and the basis for the categories of behaviour for the two schedules was taken from *Frontiers of Classroom Research* (Boydell, 1975).

The two observation schedules were devised under the headings:

> **Schedule 1: Concentration and Attention**
> **Schedule 2: Relationships and Social Interaction Analysis**.
> (See Appendix 5.)

As can be seen in Appendix 5, these schedules contained varying observation categories, such as **'Pupil situation in class'**, 'Type of activity', 'Concentration and attention' and 'Relationships and social'. For the purposes of analysis, the 'behaviour' categories under 'F' were divided into positive and negative behaviours. In Schedule 1, categories (a), (b) and (d) were rated as positive behaviours, and categories (c), (e), (f) and (g) as negative behaviours. In Schedule 2, categories (a)–(h) were rated as positive behaviours, and categories (i)–(n) and category (o) ('no interaction') were rated as negative behaviours. It can be argued that 'no interaction' is not necessarily a 'negative behaviour', but as, in this instance, we were looking for 'an increase in social interaction', it was decided that, for the purposes of this particular investigation, it should be rated as a negative behaviour.

Setting Up the Action Research Project and Collecting the Data

This project was undertaken with a group of eight 6–8-year-old children with severe learning difficulties, all of whom were able to move, run, slide and jump with ease, and who, on the whole, had a lot of collective energy! Having obtained permission from the parents and carers of the participating pupils for the children to take part in the project, there was the need for a certain amount of preparation work to be done before we could begin making the observations.

In order to lessen the time it would take to obtain an adequate number of observations, we decided that two observers would work together. This meant that before the schedules could be put to use, they had to be tested for 'reliability':

> *To be reliable... the measures would have to produce comparable estimates of children's behaviour from independent observers and yield similar scores...* (Shaffer, 1996, p. 15)

The observers also needed to familiarise themselves with and become confident with the use of the schedules, which involved recording observations at specified time intervals. Having had several practice runs, the observers were then in the position to test the 'reliability' of each of the schedules. Working from different, unobtrusive positions in the classroom, the observers recorded observations of the same child and then compared results. It was found that there was very little discrepancy, and what there was, was due to the misunderstanding of terminology. This familiarisation and test for reliability also had another advantage, in that the pupils soon became used to the presence of the observers in the classroom.

In consultation with the class teacher, it was agreed that observations would be made in two very different classroom situations. For Schedule 1 observations, the pupils would be working at set table tasks – sometimes alone, sometimes within a group, and, at other times, with the supervision and/or support of an adult. For Schedule 2 observations, the room would be organised to allow free movement from one activity to another, according to choice. Adults, also, would be free to move around in the group, as they felt appropriate. At the time the observations were being made, the adults were not aware which of the pupils were being observed.

When the observations were made immediately following a movement session, we felt it was important to ensure that pupils were observed in varying order on return to the classroom; for example, if a pupil was observed first on one occasion, then he may have been observed last on the next occasion. For the purposes of organisation, each of the pupils was given an identification number. The observers worked out a rota so that (a) they did not observe the same children each time and (b) the order of observation was rotated. It is also important to note that the observers took no part in the movement sessions. They waited in the classroom until the pupils returned from the hall.

Using the same procedure for each schedule and both the variables – 'non-Movement' and 'Movement' – observations were made of each pupil every 10 seconds over a period of 4 minutes on three occasions. This gave the following database:

Time Interval	No. of Observations per Session	Number of Occasions	Total
Every 10 seconds over 4 minutes	24	3	72

Given that there were eight pupils in the group, this gave us a theoretical possibility of 576 observations for each variable – 'non-Movement' following 'Movement' – for comparison and analysis for each of the schedules. (This number, we found, varied slightly due to the absence of particular pupils on some occasions.)

Presentation of the Results

Using Schedule 1, under 'non-Movement', a total of 528 observations were made, of which 352 were classified as positive behaviours and 176 as negative behaviours. Of the total of 552 observations made immediately following a movement session, 465 recorded positive behaviours, compared with 87 negative behaviours.

Although results from using Schedule 2 were not as numerically diverse as those from using Schedule 1, the data collected were, nonetheless, very encouraging. Out of a total of 552 observations made under 'non-Movement', totals of 201 positive behaviours and 351 negative behaviours were recorded, whereas, from a total of 560 'Movement' observations, positive behaviours increased to 305, whilst negative behaviours decreased to 255.

Accepting the suggestion that:

> *Where a single measure or a diagram can be used to present in a simple and straightforward way a concept, a pattern or a set of data, then it is usually preferable to pages of written description,* (Goulding, 1984, p. 251)

the following tables show clearly the changes within the study group, in terms of both positive and negative behaviours, following SDM sessions.

Table 9:1 Totals and Percentages for Schedule 1

Variables	No. of Observations	Positive Behaviours No.	% of Total	Negative Behaviours No.	% of Total
Non-Movement	528	352	66.7%	176	33.3%
Movement	552	465	84.2%	87	15.8%

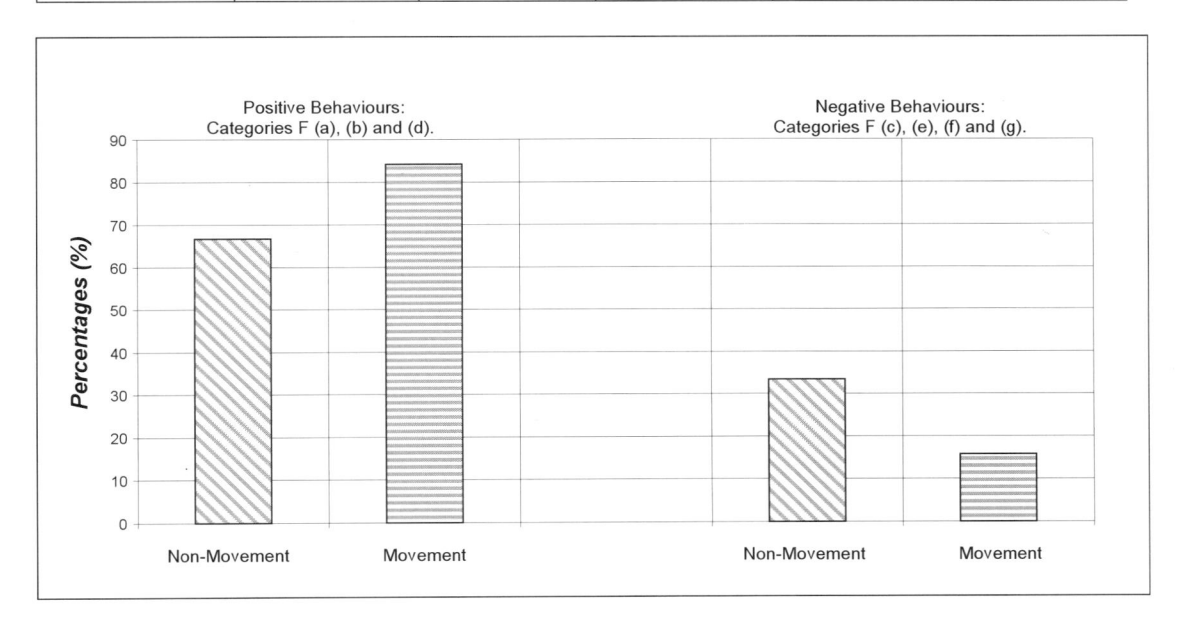

Figure 9.1: Combined Percentage Values for Positive and Negative Behaviours using Schedule 1

Table 9:2 Totals and Percentages for Schedule 2

Variables	No. of Observations	Positive Behaviours No.	% of Total	Negative Behaviours No.	% of Total
Non-Movement	552	201	36.4%	351	63.6%
Movement	560	305	54.5%	255	45.5%

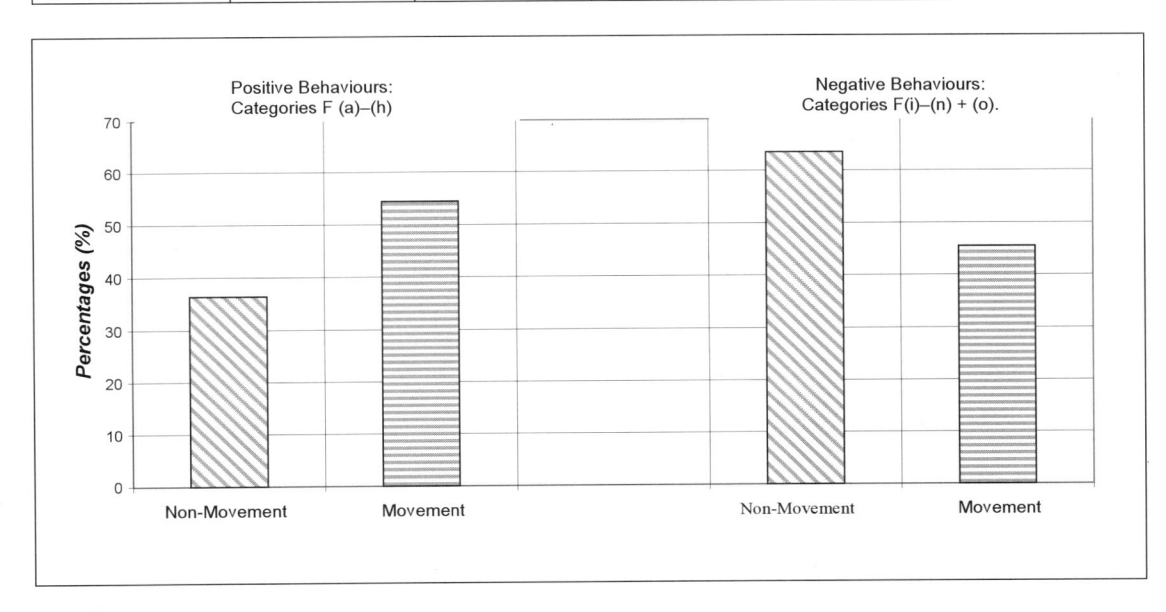

Figure 9.2 Combined Percentage Values of Positive and Negative Behaviours Using Schedule 2

Although this was a small-scale investigation and accepting that:

> ... it is likely that the size of small scale studies will be such that the results will be illuminative rather than generalizable, (Ibid., p. 230)

the results of this investigation – which centred on the effect that SDM might have on classroom behaviour in terms of concentration and attention, social interaction and, therefore, indirectly on the teaching and learning process – are very encouraging. Having said that, perhaps the *most* important bonus, which comes with the undertaking of this type of work, is the development of the very positive relationships such activities foster between the pupils and the adults working with them. An investigation which specifically focuses on the quality of the interaction between group participants and their supporting people (be they teachers, therapists, care workers, parents or any other relevant professionals) could be the subject of very meaningful, future research.

References
Boydell, D. (1975) 'Systematic observation in informal classrooms'. In: G. Chanan and F. Delamont (eds) *Frontiers of Classroom Research*. Slough: NFER.
Cohen, L. and Marion, L. (1984) 'Action research'. In: J. Bell et al. (eds) *Conducting Small Scale Investigations in Educational Management*. London: Paul Chapman/Open University.
Croll, P. (1986) *Systematic Classroom Observation*. Lewes: Falmer.
Goulding, S. (1984) 'Analysis and presentation of information'. In: J. Bell et al. (eds) *Conducting Small Scale Investigations in Educational Management*. London: Paul Chapman/Open University.
Hopkins, D. (1985) *A Teacher's Guide to Classroom Research*. Milton Keynes: Open University Press.
Shaffer D. (1996) *Developmental Psychology: Childhood and adolescence* (4th edn). Pacific Grove: Brooks/Cole Publishing Company.
Sherborne, V. (2001) *Developmental Movement for Children: Mainstream, special needs and pre-school* (2nd edn). London: Worth Publishing.

On-Going Research (1)
The classroom action research project previously described was undertaken in 1999. Accounts of two more recent research projects have been kindly contributed by research leaders, Dr Elizabeth Marsden, University of Paisley, Scotland, and Jotham Konaka, Sunfield School, Clent, West Midlands.

Dr Marsden, a founder member of The Sherborne Association UK, and its present international representative, has recently been leading a research project in a mainstream infant school in Kent, to study:

The effects of SDM in a mainstream school in England on the development of movement vocabulary and on cognitive and social milestones.

Dr Elizabeth Marsden, University of Paisley, Scotland
Sherborne (2001) made many claims for her particular style of movement education. She believed that it helped meet children's need of 'feeling at home in their own bodies'. Other authors may refer to this as developing kinaesthetic sense. She also claimed that it helped children to increase their concentration and to pay attention, as well as helping them to form relationships with each other, thus improving their social development. Much of Veronica's work was carried out in special schools, but since her movement philosophy was built on that of Rudolf Laban's work (1985), there is no reason why SDM should not benefit mainstream children as much as those in special schools. No work, to date, has been carried out to test these hypotheses amongst mainstream infant children so the University of Paisley School of Education funded the following project in a primary school in Kent during 2003–2004.

Three classes of Year 1 children were identified for this study. Classes A and B were known as the 'treatment groups' and Class C became the 'control group'. Within each group, eight females and eight males were randomly assigned as subjects (n=48). All three groups were baseline tested for development in movement, ability to concentrate and in their social development. The teacher of Class A was trained in SDM, and she taught one period of SDM to Class A and Class B for six months. Both classes also had two periods per week of traditional Physical Education (PE). Class C continued to have three periods of traditional PE taught by their own teacher.

After six months, all the children were tested again, and the results were recorded and analysed by a statistician. Results showed improvements in all areas by all three groups as would be expected through normal child development. But those children exposed to SDM showed a much bigger gain (ANOVA; p=.001) in all items relating to movement development. In fact, their gain was so great that it was **four** times greater than the control group. These results were confirmed using the non-parametric Kruskal Wallis test.

The post-treatments results for social development and ability to concentrate were equally exciting. The groups exposed to SDM improved well beyond what would be expected compared with the normal growth and development shown by the control group. Whilst the numbers in the study were small (n=48), it does go some way to show that Veronica's claims for this type of movement programme can be taken seriously.

Thanks go to the following people who helped with this study: Carrie Weston, Mario Hair, Carolyn Childs, Fiona Ong, the pupils and staff of Herne Infants School and the University of Paisley.

On-Going Research (2)
Since 2003, I have been involved in the setting up and implementation of a collaborative research project between Sunfield School in the West Midlands

and The Sherborne Association UK. The project leader is Jotham Konaka, a teacher at the school, and the project title is:

Developing social engagement through movement: exploring the perceived effectiveness of the SDM programme for children with Autistic Spectrum Disorders (ASD).

Jotham S. Konaka, Teacher, Sunfield School
SDM has been recognised as a highly effective movement programme for children and young people with special educational needs (SEN) (DES, 1991; Sherborne, 2001; Sugden and Wright, 2001). Nonetheless, the original work of the late Veronica Sherborne focused predominantly on providing movement experiences to individuals with severe learning difficulties/disabilities (Peter, 1997), physical disabilities and those who are emotionally and behaviourally disturbed. Sherborne's findings with these groups showed improved communication, greater body awareness, improved social interaction, improved development of relationships and an enhanced environmental awareness following regular sessions of SDM (Sherborne, 2001).

However, in spite of the extensive use of SDM in the context of special education needs to influence these developments, scant reference is made to those with Autistic Spectrum Disorders (ASD). Notably, at the time of SDM's inception, autism would have been less clearly defined and certainly would not have identified itself as a spectrum disorder including children so profoundly affected.

Autism has been defined as a spectrum of developmental disorders manifested in a triad of impairments characterised by a lack of social interaction, deficits in verbal and non-verbal communication, as well as rigidity of thought and behaviour (Jordan, 2002; Jordan and Powell, 2002; Wing, 1996), which adversely affects the child's educational performance. However, as Michael Guralnick (2004) suggests, 'We now know so much about childhood disability that we must move to second generation research', which focuses on problems encountered by children with autism as challenges that can be overcome through early intervention rather than deficits.

If Sherborne's claims for SDM were true for other children with special education needs, then why should a child with ASD not receive similar benefits from it? This research is based on the hypothesis that SDM has the *potential* to provide social experiences for children with profound ASD in a manner sensitive and appropriate to their individual sensory modalities and social preferences – thus building the foundations of communication. However, minimal detailed research has been carried out to explore SDM's perceived effectiveness amongst children with ASD; therefore, a collaborative research project between Sunfield School and The Sherborne Association UK has been funded by The Three Guineas Trust during 2004–2006.

The groups of children forming the basis for the study are purposive samples which do not constitute a homogenous group. The methodology reflects the individuality of each child within the cohort. The study involves six classes at Sunfield School with a total of 29 children, and ten classes in ten other UK schools which cater for children with ASD, with a total of 50 children. The groups include male and female pupils, and the age range covered is 7–19 years.

This exploratory research has adopted a case study strategy. The action research design reflects the cyclical nature of strategies employed to secure the engagement of the young people in movement experiences, as well as the evaluation of the perceived benefits accrued. Each individual case study and quasi-experiment is monitored through video analysis and naturalistic observation reports recorded at the end of each period of intervention. These observations form the basis of the planned action for the next intervention phase.

The two-year project is organised in four phases. Phase 1 (September –December 2004) involved evaluating the effectiveness and appropriateness of the existing SDM programme in relation to children with profound ASD. The researcher offered two 30-minute sessions each week, over a period of six weeks, to each of the six groups of 4–6 pupils, all with profound ASD. Each session was video taped to enable detailed analysis.

The data generated from each session was analysed against the existing SDM programme design. This allowed the researcher to identify areas of the programme which worked well as they were, and those which needed to be modified or completely changed in order to meet the needs of children with profound ASD. The programme was then adjusted, and a preliminary, revised SDM programme – specifically adapted for children with ASD – was produced.

Phase 2 (February–October 2005) involved working with two other schools to fine tune the revised SDM programme. The revised programme was trialled initially at Sunfield and in two other schools for children with ASD. Again, video observations informed the process, and analysis by the researcher identified any need for modifications to the programme (September–October 2005).

During the programme implementation at Phase 3 (November 2005–February 2006), the revised SDM programme for children with ASD was given to 10 schools for children with ASD. Teachers were asked to use the programme during 30-minute SDM sessions, at least twice weekly, keeping notes at the end of each lesson on the effectiveness of the activities. Two visits to each research school by the researcher to offer support and advice occurred during the period. The researcher also continued focused work at Sunfield, and video records were kept and analysed against the trial programme. Phase 4 (March–September 2006) will involve project evaluation and writing the final programme, as well as designing and editing a video.

The project findings and revised SDM (ASD) programme will be disseminated through Sunfield Professional Development Centre training, the Sunfield website (www.sunfield-school.org.uk), professional journals, a video and through The Sherborne Association UK.

References

Department of Education and Science (1991) *National Curriculum Physical Education for Ages 5–6*. London: HMSO.

Guralnick, M. (2004) 'Early intervention for children with intellectual disabilities: current knowledge and future prospects'. Paper presented at the 12th IASSID World Congress, Montpellier, France (June).

Jordan, R. (1999) *Autistic Spectrum Disorders: An introductory handbook for practitioners*. London: David Fulton.

Jordan, R. and Powell, S. (1995) *Understanding and Teaching Children with Autism*. Chichester: John Wiley.

Laban, R. (1975) *Principles of Dance and Movement Notation*. London: MacDonald.

Peter, M. (1997) *Making Dance Special*. London: David Fulton.

Sherborne, V. (2001) *Developmental Movement for Children: Mainstream, special needs and pre-school (2nd edition)*. London: Worth Publishing.

Sherborne Association (2002) 'Teaching notes and guidelines'. Available through The Sherborne Association UK (www.sherborne-association.org.uk).

Sugden, D. and Wright, H. (2001) 'Physical Education'. In: B. Carpenter, R. Ashdown and K. Bovair (eds) *Enabling Access: Effective teaching and learning for pupils with learning difficulties*. London: David Fulton.

Wing, L. (1996) *The Autistic Spectrum: A guide for parents and professionals. Suffolk*: St. Edmunsbury Press.

*Reprinted by kind permission of Worth Publishing from *Developmental Movement for Children* by Veronica Sherborne. 2nd Edition. Worth Publishing Limited 2001.

CHAPTER 10
A Concluding Summary

It could be argued that the main title of this work, *Communicating through Movement*, is too broad a concept for a book that has focused on a specific method and way of working. However, 'communication', at varying levels, is something that is intrinsic to all aspects of Sherborne's work. Whilst the first part of the subtitle, *Sherborne Developmental Movement*, directs the reader towards the subject of its contents, the latter part, *towards a broadening perspective*, reflects the way in which the work has developed, and its use extended, over recent years.

From its early beginnings in the mid-1950s, Sherborne Developmental Movement (SDM) has evolved into a way of working that, from its early conception in which Sherborne used her ideas with students as a means of helping them 'to work together and feel secure within the group', until the present time, has been valued and implemented internationally, across a broad spectrum of professions and needs. That the work is used in education, in the care professions, by psychologists and therapists bears testimony to its versatility, accessibility and lasting value.

In her films and videos, the last of which was *Good Companions* (see Appendix 6), and in her book, *Developmental Movement for Children*, Sherborne has left us a clearly defined practical structure for her work, in which she describes, and in some cases illustrates with photographs, many of the 'experiences' in her movement repertoire, interspersed with brief personal observations concerning the theoretical and philosophical framework of SDM, and the benefits her work has to offer children with varying special needs.

In order to help us to understand Sherborne's work, it is important that we have an awareness of its roots. From the biographical knowledge we have of Veronica Sherborne, it is obvious that, from the outset, she was drawn towards a vocation which brought her into contact with 'the more vulnerable members of society'. Her work at the Withymead Centre in Devon spanned a period of 15 years, during which time her interest broadened, through her early work with students, to include work with children who were at that time referred to as 'mentally handicapped'. Following Sherborne's own book, *Developmental Movement for Children*, which must always remain the definitive document for her work, it is my hope that in this book I have offered 'a broadening perspective' which encompasses the use of her ideas by users and enthusiasts across an expanding spectrum of environments and professions.

For students who become involved in an academic study of the work, I have included references which are aimed at substantiating some of the claims made by Sherborne concerning beneficial aspects of using her ideas, along with an investigation into the philosophical modalities and 'evolving theory' which underpin her work. The way we present Sherborne Development Movement, in whatever context, is crucial to its successful implementation and, for those who are about to embark on its use or who may already be using Sherborne's ideas, I hope that the sections of the book which have focused on practice will be both helpful and supportive.

Research into SDM there must be if the work is to move forward from a solid, substantiated foundation. I hope that the accounts of recent research projects will make some contribution towards inspiring more in the future.

Although its genesis was in the field of special education in the UK, SDM is being used quite extensively both in the therapeutic setting and in therapy both in the UK and abroad. Sherborne always insisted that her work was not a 'therapy'. She was quite adamant about this, and rightly so. There is a clear distinction between 'therapy', where the work is undertaken by fully trained, qualified therapists, and a situation where the work may well be considered to have a 'therapeutic' effect on the participants. Sherborne considered her work as belonging to the latter of these categories. There is no doubt that her work, when implemented successfully, does have a 'therapeutic effect' and can contribute towards a feeling of 'well-being' for those who are involved in it.

Combining, as they do, both physiological and psychological learning experiences, all these examples of the 'broadening perspective' in which Sherborne's ideas are now being applied support her definition of the movements as 'experiences' rather then 'exercises'. There is no doubt that, in all of the situations described above, involvement in SDM can have a considerable psychological effect on the participants. SDM can be a powerful 'tool' offering much towards personal development and a developing awareness of the feelings and needs of others.

Finally, in bringing this book to its conclusion, I am going to be totally subjective! I personally have no doubts whatsoever as to the benefits of Sherborne's way of working. For me, the philosophy which underpins it has become a way of life. For me, it is of the utmost importance that when engaged in work which involves close contact with other people, be it physically, intellectually, emotionally or socially, the prime consideration should centre around a way forward for everyone involved, in a positive atmosphere created within an ethos of 'success' based on shared movement experiences. That is not to say that we should become patronising. It is not to say that we should 'pretend' that everything is right and correct. What it does mean is that when changes need to be made through SDM, be they intellectual or cognitive in terms of the learning process, or developmental in terms of personal attributes or self-concept, then attempts to implement those changes are made according to individual needs and supported by 'constructive suggestion' within an atmosphere which is non-judgemental and inclusive. To me, Sherborne's work can offer so much in so many different ways, and I hope this has been highlighted within this book. However, the true value and quality of Sherborne's work can be appreciated fully only through doing it and becoming involved in its implementation.

Reading a book, as valuable as that may be, is not enough in itself if the work is to continue to be maintained in the future.

Earlier in this 'Concluding Summary', I used the word 'enthusiast'. I used that word deliberately. During my conversations with Sherborne colleagues both in the UK and in many other countries, 'enthusiasm' and 'excitement' are very appropriate words to describe the emotions that accompany those conversations. We must not be afraid or reticent about sharing this enthusiasm with others. I know it can be very challenging when asked a question such as, 'What is it all about – "this cradling", "curling up", "bound flow", etc.?', by someone who is not familiar with the work. However, my sincere hope is that this book may make some contribution towards making those questions less intimidating, whilst at the same time, in a professional setting, providing a degree of awareness and knowledge which will facilitate meaningful discussion, undertaken not only with enthusiasm, but also with an appreciable degree of confidence.

In terms of the work itself, I have learnt not to expect too much too soon! There can be no hard and fast rules about how a session will develop or how participants will respond. That is the joy and excitement of the work which will come with experience of both session leaders and participants.

It is essential to remember that the *'evolving theory'* referred to in Part 1 is exactly that, and has come about through interpretation of Sherborne's own writings, and deliberations and discussions between people who, over a period of time, worked closely with her. The work is still open, to a great extent, to 'personal interpretation'. As Sherborne says in the summary of her book, 'each teacher or caregiver can make use of the material described in this book in his or her own way'*. The interpretation of the ethos of SDM by practitioners *must* remain subjective, but needs to be backed up and substantiated by research and an awareness of the theory and philosophy that underpins the work. It has been my intention in this book to address both of those equally important aspects.

In conclusion, it has to be acknowledged that, as with much work of this kind, SDM may not be suitable for everyone. However, given an awareness of the underlying theory and philosophy, an acceptance of the teaching styles, the approach necessary for its implementation, and regular sessions over a reasonable period of time, then, in the vast majority of cases, 'It works!' Moreover, with a considerable degree of confidence, we can also begin to understand *Why* it works.

APPENDIX 1
Sherborne Developmental Movement

Two basic objectives

1. Awareness of self   **2. Awareness of others**

Awareness of self

Body awareness   Spatial awareness

Confidence in self
and a positive self-image

Awareness of others

Relationships
(with a partner/in a group)

'with/caring'   'shared'   'against'

Trust and confidence
in self and others

Creativity and a developing awareness of varying movement
qualities are constant themes throughout all movement activities.

APPENDIX 2
Developing Relationships

Underpinning all relationship work is the development of trust and confidence in self and others. In movement terms these relationships fall into 'three broad categories'.

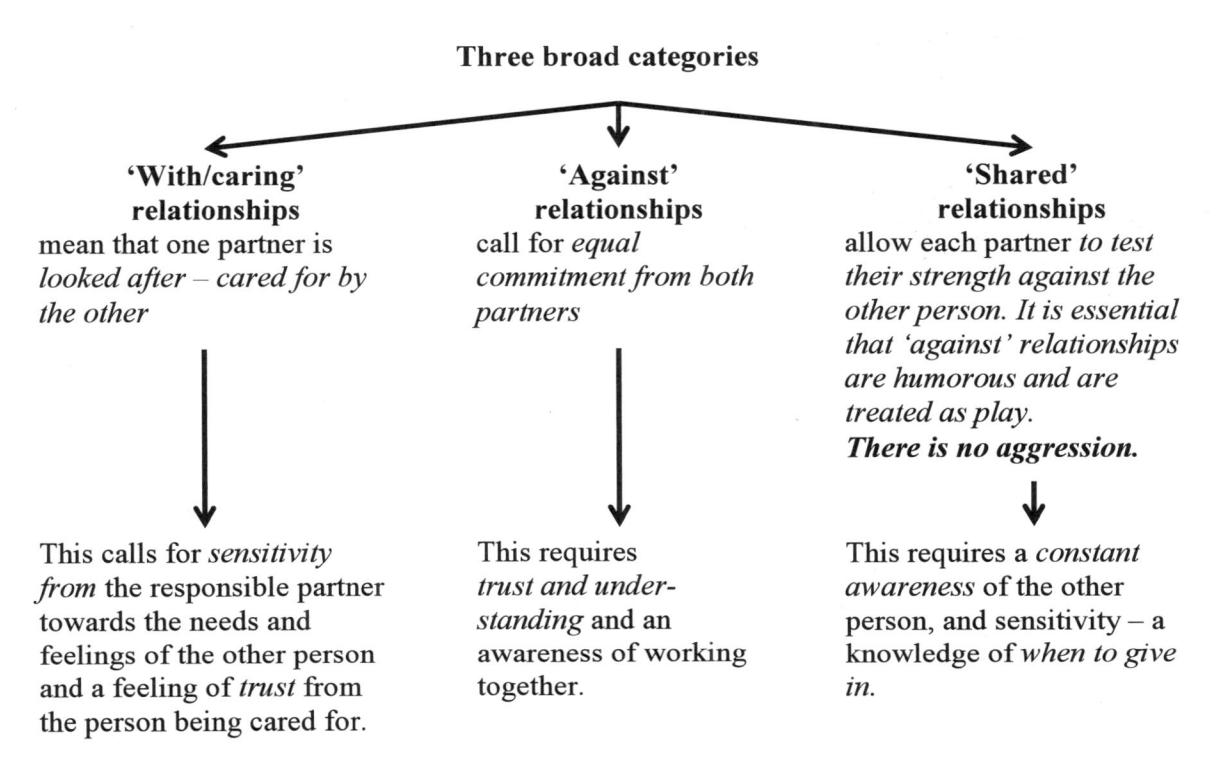

Three broad categories

'With/caring' relationships	'Against' relationships	'Shared' relationships
mean that one partner is *looked after – cared for by the other*	call for *equal commitment from both partners*	allow each partner *to test their strength against the other person. It is essential that 'against' relationships are humorous and are treated as play.* **There is no aggression.**
This calls for *sensitivity from* the responsible partner towards the needs and feelings of the other person and a feeling of *trust* from the person being cared for.	This requires *trust and understanding* and an awareness of working together.	This requires a *constant awareness* of the other person, and sensitivity – a knowledge of *when to give in.*

Examples of the potential to generalise from the three types of relationships experienced in SDM:

- **With relationships**
  These can help to develop an understanding of **turn-taking** and **decision-making,** such as when to change roles

- **Shared relationships**
  These can help to develop an understanding of **equality** – a co-operative type of behaviour **with equal responsibility.**

- **Against relationships**
  These can help to develop the feeling of a sustained effort – the ability to **concentrate**.

<u>**Erratum: Page 127**</u>
Two of the second-level diagram headings – **'Against' relationships** and **'Shared' relationships** – which appear immediately below the first level diagram heading, **Three broad categories**, should be transposed.

APPENDIX 3
Sherborne Developmental Movement Experiences Presented in Four Progressive Stages

STAGE ONE

1. Activities

1.1. Body Awareness

Floor-Based

1.1.1. *Hips*
Sliding, shuffling on hips

1.1.2. *Stomach*
Wriggling on stomach – encourage movement

1.1.3. *Back*
Wriggling on back – forwards/backwards/side to side

1.1.4. *Centres*
Curling up

In Sitting Position

1.1.5. *Knees*
Make knees appear/disappear, pat, rub, tickle, thump

1.1.6. *Elbows*
Make elbows appear/disappear, pat, rub, tickle, thump

1.1.7. *Feet*
Slap feet on floor, circle feet in the air

1.1.8. *Arms*
Straighten, bend, shake arms

1.1.9. *Hands*
Clap, shake hands

Standing

1.1.10. *Legs*
Walking, running – with big steps, little steps

1.1.11. *Whole Body*
  i. Rolling
  ii. Make body wide/straight/long/small

1.1.12. *Falling*
From side onto back or front

1.2. Spatial Awareness

1.2.1. *Personal Space/Lying on Back/Sitting and Standing*
Explore space above and to the side, using arms and legs

1.2.2. *General Space*
Walking, running – stop, start

1.3. Relationships

'With' Relationships

1.3.1. *Back-to-Back*
Wriggling/pushing against each other's back

1.3.2. *Back-to-Back Slide*
One partner *pushing* the other partner along the floor

1.3.3. *Cradling/Rocking*
Partners sit one behind the other; person behind places hands on partner's shoulders – rock gently

1.3.4. *Rolling*
Roll partner away from you

1.3.5. *Rolling*
Roll partner towards you

'Against' Relationships

1.3.6. *Back-to-Back*
Pushing – testing strength

'Shared' Relationships

- **1.3.7.** *Back-to-Back*
  Relaxing against partner's back – sway together

- **1.3.8.** *Sitting Facing Each Other*
  Hold hands – move and sway together

1.4. Group Work

- **1.4.1.** *Holding Hands in Circle*
  Move forwards/sideways/backwards – sit down in close group

STAGE TWO

2. Activities

2.1. Body Awareness

Floor-Based

- **2.1.1.** *Hips*
  Bumping, spinning on hips

- **2.1.2.** *Stomach*
  Sliding on stomach, pulling with arms

- **2.1.3.** *Back*
  Sliding on back, pushing with feet

- **2.1.4.** *Centre*
  Alternate curling up and stretching out

In Sitting Position

- **2.1.5.** *Knees/Elbows*
  Knock knees with elbows:
  i. right elbow – right knee
  ii. left elbow – left knee
  iii. left elbow – right knee
  iv. right elbow – left knee

- **2.1.6.** *Feet*
  Tap toes on floor, slap balls of feet on floor, drum heels on floor

2.1.7. *Arms*
Stretch arms:
i. high above head
ii. both out to one side
iii. out to both sides
iv. fold across body

2.1.8. *Hands*
Stretch/clench

2.1.9. *Face*
Make:
i. eyes – big/small
ii. mouth – big/small
iii. whole face – big/small

In Standing Position

2.1.10. *Legs*
Walk:
i. from side to side
ii. forwards/backwards

2.1.11. *Whole Body*
Bend trunk:
i. from side to side
ii. forwards/backwards

Lying on Floor

2.1.12. *Rolling*
With whole body:
i. stiff/floppy
ii. quickly/slowly

Sitting Cross-Legged on Floor

2.1.13. *Falling*
Rocking movement – weight on thighs, upper arm, elbow – roll onto back, roll onto side, push up on upper arm and elbow, back into sitting position; stay curled up throughout

2.2. Spatial Awareness

Personal Space

2.2.1. *In Sitting Position*
Using arms and legs – explore space in front, to both sides and behind

General Space

2.2.2. *Walking/Running*
  i. start/stop 'high' – arms reaching above head
  ii. start/stop 'low' – crouched

2.2.3. *Moving towards Selected Spot*
  i. sliding on stomachs (low)
  ii. shuffling on hips (medium)
  iii. walking/running (eye level) – move directly/flexibly

2.2.4. *Spatial Concepts*
See 'with' relationships, 2.3.9

2.3. Relationships

'With' Relationships

2.3.1. *Supporting/Balancing – Back-to-Back*
Supporter bends forwards – partner leans on offered back

2.3.2. *Supporter on All Fours*
Other partner lies across supporter's back on stomach; hands and feet on floor

2.3.3. Other partner sits on supporter's hips, facing *forwards* – lies on stomach along partner's back

2.3.4. Other partner sits on supporter's hips, facing *backwards* – lies on back along partner's back

2.3.5. *Trust*
One partner lies on back stretched 'wide' – other partner steps over body/arms/legs

2.3.6. *Sliding*
Pushing partner from behind using feet/hands/shoulders/head

2.3.7. *Cradling/Rocking*
Supporter sits behind partner, hands on partner's shoulders – partner leans back against supporter whilst gently being rocked

2.3.8. *Rolling*
Roll partner away from you using feet

2.3.9. *Spatial Concepts*
Make a shape for your partner to crawl/slide through/under

2.4. Group Work

2.4.1. *In a Circle*
Tie group into a 'knot' – everyone move towards the centre, weave in and out without letting go of hands, sit down

2.4.2. *Tunnels*
Small groups make tunnels for other people to crawl through

2.4.3. *Tunnels*
Whole group makes long tunnel – end person crawls/slides through, followed by next person; when end of tunnel is reached, join on to front of tunnel, so that tunnel moves towards a pre-selected spot

STAGE THREE

3. Activities

3.1. Body Awareness

3.1.1. *Hips*
i. walking on hips, backwards/forwards
ii. rocking on hips sideways
iii. sequence of movements – spin/roll/spin...

3.1.2. *Stomach*
Spinning on stomach, hands and feet off floor – slap hands on floor to push

3.1.3. *Back*
Spin on backs – use hands and feet to propel

3.1.4. *Centres*
Curling and stretching – fast/slow (vary speed)

3.1.5. *Combine Legs/Elbows/Centres*
'Lizard' creeping – right knee touches right elbow, left knee touches left elbow – encourage flexibility at waist

3.1.6. *Knees*
i. walking on knees – forwards/backwards/sideways
ii. introduce smaller parts of body – chin on knee, nose on knee, finger on knee, thumbs on knees, etc.

In Sitting Position

3.1.7. *Ankles*
Lift feet off floor – make circular up and down and side to side movements with ankles

3.1.8. *Wrists*
Arms stretched out – make circular up and down and side to side movements from wrists

Standing

3.1.9. *Whole Body*
From a sitting position, rock backwards and forwards on shoulders – try to touch floor behind head with feet, rock up onto hips, back onto shoulders, etc.

3.1.10. *Falling*
From kneeling on all fours – ***tuck head in***, fall forwards onto forearm, then shoulder, roll onto back; ***keep curled up***, continue rolling on into all fours position

3.2. Spatial Awareness

3.2.1. *Personal Space*
In standing position:
i. explore space – in front, to the side, above and below, behind; using arms, legs and trunk, introduce 'twist' to see 'behind'
ii. explore space 'behind' by stepping backwards, putting hands on floor, then lifting one leg 'up' and 'behind'

3.2.2. *General Space*
Walking/running – stop/start, change direction, move backwards/forwards

3.2.3. *High Space*
Focus on a high spot – run, then jump towards it

3.2.4. *Behind*
Focus on spot 'behind' – run away from it; jump, turning towards it; run towards it

3.2.5. *Spatial Concepts*
See 'With' Relationships, 3.3.11.

3.3. Relationships

'With' Relationships

3.3.1. *Trust*
One partner lies on the floor spread out 'wide' – other partner walks/jumps over arms/legs/body

3.3.2. *Supporting and Balance – Back-to-Back*
Supporter leans forwards – partner slides shoulders up supporter's back; raises hips off floor

3.3.3. *Supporting on Back*
Supporting partner kneels on all fours – other partner lies on stomach on supporter's back; lifts feet off floor

3.3.4. *Forward Sliding*
Partners sitting one behind the other – rear partner slides other partner forwards by shuffling on hips

3.3.5. *Slides*
One partner lies on back or stomach – other partner pulls them along by arms or legs

3.3.6. *Cradling/Rocking*
Supporting partner 'contains' other partner with arms and legs – contained partner curls up and is rocked gently

3.3.7. *Face-to-Face Rocking*
Partners sit facing each other – lean forward; rest heads on each other's shoulders; rock together

3.3.8. *Taking Partner for a Walk*
One partner makes body strong; other partner makes theirs 'floppy' – strong partner takes floppy partner for a supported walk

3.3.9. *Rolling*
Roll partner towards you using heels

3.3.10. *Flexibility at Waist and Relaxation*
i. one partner lies on side, hands above head – other partner puts hands on shoulder and hip, gently twists trunk by pushing shoulder forwards and hip back, then shoulder back and hip forwards, alternately, to get flexibility and relaxation at waist, *then*
ii. gently pushes or pulls partner so that he/she falls onto back or stomach

3.3.11. *Spatial Concepts*
i. on/over – one partner makes body shapes for other partner to rest 'on' or climb 'over'
ii. In/out – one partner is contained by other partner – 'friendly' battle to get 'out'; runs away; at signal, runs back to partner to be contained ('in')

'Against' Relationships

3.3.12. *Limpets*
One partner, lying either on front or back, 'sticks' to the floor – other partner attempts to upset or turn over the prone or supine partner who will resist

'Shared' Relationships

3.3.13. *Shared Rolling*
Both partners lie on stomachs on the floor, head to head, holding hands – roll together, forwards and backwards

3.3.14. *See-Saw*
Partners stand holding hands – one partner crouches; standing partner pulls other upright, then crouches; alternate movement creates see-saw motion

3.3.15. *Rowing*
Partners sit facing each other holding hands – one partner lies back until head touches floor and is then pulled up by other partner; roles reverse as 'pulling' partner lies back until head touches floor

3.3.16. *Balanced Standing*
Partners stand facing each other, holding hands – both lean back until arms are straight; both go down into crouched position, then move back to standing, keeping arms straight all the time

3.4. Group Work

3.4.1. Group Supporting
Three/four/five people go onto all fours, side by side, with shoulder and hips touching; one person lies along backs on stomach or back – group can rock or move forwards/backwards/sideways/up and down

3.4.2. 'A Pile of People'
Everyone moves on hips towards centre of room – all sit as close together as possible, then lie back; people on the outside move away first, then can pull others away from the pile

STAGE FOUR

4. Activities

4.1. Body Awareness

4.1.1. Legs/Knees
Walk with 'high' knees – allow 'high' knees to lead and change direction

4.1.2. 'Little' Legs
In crouched position, hands on knees:
  i. walk with knees stuck together/wide apart/forwards/backwards/sideways
  ii. jump – forwards/sideways/backwards

4.1.3. Whole Body/Trunk – Open/Closed Rolling
When on back, *curl up*, when on stomach, *stretch out*

4.1.4. Open/Closed Sliding
Lying on stomach – pull up onto knees and forearms, stretch out; repeat

4.1.5. Flexible Rolling
  i. lead with shoulders, hips follow
  ii. lead with hips, shoulders follow, producing 'twist' and flexibility at waist

4.1.6. Falling
  i. from standing – jump into crouched position; go onto all fours; follow sequence as in Stage 3
  ii. from running – jump into crouched position; follow sequence as in Stage 3

4.2. Spatial Awareness

Personal Space

4.2.1. *From Standing*
Develop concept of personal space as a 'sphere/bubble/ball'; introduce notion of *moving* 'bubble' around in the environment using varying movement qualities; for example, bubble filled with:
i. not-quite-set concrete – slow, heavy movements
ii. feathers – light, flicking movements
iii. treacle – slow, flowing movements (hands and feet 'stuck' together, having to be drawn apart)
iv. rubber – strong, quick, bouncing movements

4.2.2. Explore possible *size* and *shape* of bubble:
i. open – arms and legs extended, body in open attitude
ii. closed – arms and legs crossed over the body
iii. high/big – reaching as high as possible
iv. low/small – crouch close to the floor

Move around in varying combinations; for example, high/open, low/closed, low/open – encourage participants to develop own sequences

General Space

4.2.3. Run, leap, change direction in mid-air, stop high/low – encourage participants to develop own sequences

4.2.4. *Spatial concepts*
See 'With' Relationships, 4.3.3

4.3. Relationships

'With' Relationships

4.3.1. *Backwards Sitting Slides*
Partners sit one behind the other; rear partner grips with knees and locks feet under calves of front partner – slides/shuffles backwards on hips, taking partner with him/her

4.3.2. *Trust*
As in Stage 3 (3.3.1), but active partner moves around room jumping over other people, returning to own partner, pretending to be very 'fierce'

4.3.3. *Spatial Concepts*
i. in front – partners stand one 'in front' of the other, both facing the same way; the partner at the back tries to get 'in front'; the front partner dodges to try to stop him/her succeeding
ii. behind – partners stand facing each other; each tries to stop the other getting 'behind'

4.3.4. *Flexible Slide*
One partner pulls the other by arms or legs, swaying him/her from side to side, encouraging flexibility at the waist; this can also be done with partner lying on a blanket

4.3.5. *Supporting and Balancing on the Back*
Supporting partner on hands and knees, low to the floor, making back into a level platform – supported partner positions him/herself on partner's back, shoulders to shoulders, hips to hips; supporting partner comes up onto all fours, taking full body weight when partner's feet come up off the floor (can rest feet on supporting partner's heels)

4.3.6. *Shin Balance*
Supporting partner lies on back, with knees raised, presenting a platform with his/her shins for the other partner to lie on face down – supporting partner will offer stability by holding the shoulders of the supported partner

4.3.7. *Leading 'Visually Impaired' Partner*
One partner closes eyes – other partner takes 'visually impaired' partner for a walk, looking after them

'With/Against' Sequence

4.3.8.
One partner lies on the floor stretched out – the other partner gently wraps them up into a 'parcel' ('with' relationship); they then attempt to unwrap the 'parcel', who resists ('against' relationship)

'Against/Shared' Sequence

4.3.9. Partners stand or sit facing each other – push against each other's hands/feet; at an agreed point, this changes to a mirroring activity, with partners taking it in turns to lead

'Shared' Relationships

4.3.10. *Face-to-Face Rocking*
Partners sit facing each other, 'containing' each other – rock gently together

4.3.11. *Back-to-Back Standing*
Partners sit back-to-back – pushing against each other, they stand up/crouch down/stand up

4.3.12. *Upside-Down Balance*
Partners balance on shoulders, with hands and forearms on the floor, feet touching

4.4. Group Work

4.4.1. *Jumping in Threes*
Person in the middle is helped to 'jump high' (requires co-ordinated movements and support)

4.4.2. *Rocking in Threes*
Supporters sit either side of third person, supporting their head and shoulders; person in middle should support own back and sit up straight – person in middle is gently rocked from side to side

4.4.3. *Balanced Standing*
In threes/fours/fives/.../whole group – all participants join hands in a circle, lean backwards; keeping arms straight and balancing group's weight, crouch down, stand up together

4.4.4. *Slithering/Rolling on Bodies*
Group lies on floor on backs close together; one person lies along backs – as group rolls in synchrony, person is propelled along

4.4.5. *Body Push*
Group makes a small circle with one person standing in the middle – person is gently pushed around the circle, from one supporter to another, whilst keeping feet anchored to floor

4.4.6. *Tunnels/Bridges*
These can be made by any number of people and can vary in height and direction for individuals to climb/slither/slide/crawl through or over

APPENDIX 4
Sherborne Developmental Movement Assessment Procedure

It is expected that users of this assessment procedure will have undertaken SDM training, or will be working in co-operation with a person who has experience of using SDM.

Key to recording

Level of prompt/intervention

- **E**   Experiental involvement with total physical support
- **P**   Physical prompt – passive movement
- **G**   Gestural prompt – imitated movement
- **V**   Verbal prompt only
- **I**   Initiates movement

This method of recording is suitable for all participants regardless of age, gender or degree of disability.

This is one suggested way of completing the assessment; however, you may wish to substitute your own 'key to recording'.

Within the assessment procedure please read:

1. *'Participant'* as someone for whom the session has been devised and who is being assessed
2. *'Supporter'* as someone who is taking part in a supporting role.

Copyright has been waived for this assessment procedure.

Sherborne Developmental Movement Assessment Procedure
Assessment Sheet 1: Body Awareness

Overall Period of Assessment

Name: . . . .   Dates: . . . .

1. Mobility

		Date		
1.1	Moves/slides on stomach			
1.2	Moves/slides on back			
1.3	Rolls			
1.4	Walks			
1.5	Runs			
1.6	Jumps			
1.7	Gets out of wheelchair			
1.8	Gets into wheelchair			

2. Body Awareness

		Can identify (Date)			Can touch and name (Date)		
2.1	Hips						
2.2	Front of body						
2.3	Back of body						
2.4	Head						
2.5	Face						
2.6	Arms						
2.7	Hands						
2.8	Elbows						
2.9	Legs						
2.10	Knees						
2.11	Feet						
2.12	Other finer parts of body, e.g. eyes, nose, etc.						

Sherborne Developmental Movement Assessment Procedure
Assessment Sheet 1A: Body Awareness *(Ctd)*

Overall Period of Assessment

Name: .... Dates: ....

3. Centre of the Body

		Can identify			Can touch and name		
		Date			Date		
3.1	Centre of body						

		Date		
3.2	Can curl up			
3.3	Can remain curled up against resistance			

4. Spine and Trunk

		Date		
4.1	Has mobility of the spine and trunk (as in curling up and/or somersaulting)			

5. Summary of Skills in Each Area

5.1	Mobility	
5.2	Body parts	
5.3	Centre of body	
5.4	Spine and trunk	

6. Summary of Needs in Each Area

6.1	Mobility	
6.2	Body parts	
6.3	Centre of body	
6.4	Spine and trunk	

Sherborne Developmental Movement Assessment Procedure
Assessment Sheet 2: Spatial Awareness

Overall Period of Assessment

Name:........................ Dates: ....

1. Personal Space

		In lying position	In sitting position	In standing position
		Date	Date	Date
1.1	Can indicate, using arms and legs, extent of personal space			

		In sitting position		Standing
		Using feet	Using hands	Using hands and feet
		Date	Date	Date
1.2	Can 'share' personal space with a partner			

		From sitting position		From standing
		Using feet	Using hands	Using hands and feet
		Date	Date	Date
1.3	Can 'defend' personal space when working with a partner			

2. General Space

		With 'direct' movements	With 'flexible' movements
		Date	Date
2.1	Can move freely through space		

Sherborne Developmental Movement Assessment Procedure
Assessment Sheet 2A: Spatial Awareness *(Ctd)*

Overall Period of Assessment

Name: .... Dates: ....

2. General Space *(Ctd)*

2.2	Can indicate:	From sitting position Date			From standing position Date		
	in front						
	behind						
	high						
	low						
	side						
	the other side						

3. Summary of Skills in Each Area

3.1	Personal space	
3.2	General space	

4. Summary of Needs in Each Area

4.1	Personal space	
4.2	General space	

Sherborne Developmental Movement Assessment Procedure
Assessment Sheet 3: Relationships

Overall Period of Assessment

Name: .... Dates: ....

1. Joining the Group

		Supported by a supporter			Independent		
		Date			Date		
1.1	Will join a group SDM situation						

		Working with a supporter			Working with another participant		
		Date			Date		
1.2	Is able to accept back-to-back relationship						
1.3	Is able to accept face-to-face relationship						

2. 'With' Relationships

		Working with a supporter			Working with another participant		
		Date			Date		
2.1	Will allow partner to push, pull or slide him/her (specify)						
2.2	Is able to push, pull or slide a partner (specify)						
2.3	Will allow partner to support his/her weight						
2.4	Is able to support his/her partner's weight	■	■	■			

Sherborne Developmental Movement Assessment Procedure
Assessment Sheet 3A: Relationships *(Ctd)*

Overall Period of Assessment

Name: .... Dates: ....

2. 'With' Relationships *(Ctd)*

		Working with a supporter	Working with another participant
		Date	Date
2.5	Will relax when being rocked and contained		
2.6	Can contain and rock another person		
2.7	Shows sensitivity towards needs and feelings of partner		

3. 'Shared' Relationships

		Working with a supporter	Working with another participant
		Date	Date
3.1	Understands the concept of 'balanced'		
3.2	Understands the concept of 'turn-taking'		
3.3	Shows sensitivity to needs and feelings of partner		

4. 'Against' Relationships

		Working with a supporter	Working with another participant
		Date	Date
4.1	Can resist being 'uncurled'		
4.2	Can stay curled up whilst being given a slide		
4.3	Can remain curled up whilst being lifted		

Sherborne Developmental Movement Assessment Procedure
Assessment Sheet 3B: Relationships *(Ctd)*

Overall Period of Assessment

Name: …………………… Dates: ……………………………

4. 'Against' Relationships (*Ctd*)

		Working with a supporter	Working with another participant
		Date	Date
4.4	Understands concept of remaining strong against efforts to pull or push him/her over		
4.5	Understands concept of trying to pull or push another person over		
4.6	Understands concept of 'strength <u>without</u> aggression'		
4.7	Understands concept of mutual agreement on 'when to give in'		
4.8	Shows sensitivity towards needs and feelings of partner		

5. Group Work

		Mixed group of supporters and participants	Group of participants
		Date	Date
5.1	Can work co-operatively in groups of three or more people (specify)		

Sherborne Developmental Movement Assessment Procedure
Assessment Sheet 3C: Relationships *(Ctd)*

Overall Period of Assessment

Name: . . . .   Dates: . . . .

6. Summary of Observations Concerning 'Relationships' Activities Skills

6.1	'With' relationships	
6.2	'Shared' relationships	
6.3	'Against' relationships	
6.4	'Group' work	

7. Summary of Observations Concerning 'Relationships' Activities Needs

7.1	'With' relationships	
7.2	'Shared' relationships	
7.3	'Against' relationships	
7.4	'Group' work	

Sherborne Developmental Movement Assessment Procedure
Assessment Sheet 4: Movement Quality and Creativity

Overall Period of Assessment

Name:........................ Dates: ....

1. Movement Quality

	In movement terms, understands the concept of:		Date			Date		
1.1	Weight	Heavy						
		Light						
1.2	Time	Fast						
		Slow						
1.3	Movement in space	Direct						
		Flexible						
1.4	Flow of movement	Bound						
		Free						

Sherborne Developmental Movement Assessment Procedure

Assessment Sheet 4A: Movement Quality and Creativity *(Ctd)*

Name: ....

Dates: ....   Overall Period of Assessment ....

2. Creativity

		Working with an adult	Working independently	Working with another child	Working in a group
		Date	Date	Date	Date
2.1	Indicates interest in exploring space in all its dimensions				
2.2	Indicates interest in exploring different ways of executing movements				
2.3	Indicates a willingness to 'experiment' with varying movement qualities				
2.4	Can create simple sequences of movement				

APPENDIX 5
An Evaluation of Certain Aspects of Sherborne Developmental Movement

Classroom Observation Schedule (1)

Observations should be made over a 4-minute period, and recorded every 10 seconds to give 24 observations per pupil per observation period.

CONCENTRATION AND ATTENTION SKILLS

Observation Schedule Key
Pupil, Class and Observation Timing Information
A. Pupil identification number
B. Class identification
C. Observation timing:
   'M' = immediately following a Sherborne Developmental Movement (SDM) session
   'N/M' = not following an SDM session

Pupil Observation Record

D. Pupil situation in class:
   a = group – supervised
   b = group – unsupervised
   c = with peer – supervised
   d = with peer – unsupervised
   e = individual – supervised
   f = individual – unsupervised

E. Type of activity:
   a = play
   b = directed
   c = directed/choice of two
   d = free choice

F. Concentration and attention:
   a = behaving in a co-operative way
   b = staying within activity situation
   c = requiring verbal reinforcement to maintain attention
   d = changing activity with permission
   e = changing activity without permission
   f = constantly fidgeting
   g = preoccupied

A	B	C

Times (m/s)	D	E	F
0/0			
0/10			
0/20			
0/30			
0/40			
0/50			
1/0			
1/10			
1/20			
1/30			
1/40			
1/50			
2/0			
2/10			
2/20			
2/30			
2/40			
2/50			
3/0			
3/10			
3/20			
3/30			
3/40			
3/50			
4/0			

Classroom Observation Schedule (2)

Observations should be made over a 4-minute period, and recorded every 10 seconds to give 24 observations per pupil per observation period.

RELATIONSHIPS AND SOCIAL INTERACTION ANALYSIS

Observation Schedule Key
Pupil, Class and Observation Timing Information

A	B	C

A. Pupil identification number
B. Class identification
C. Observation timing:
   'M' = immediately following an SDM session
   'N/M' = not following an SDM session

Pupil Observation Record

D. Pupil situation in class:
   a = group – supervised
   b = group – unsupervised
   c = with peer – supervised
   d = with peer – unsupervised
   e = individual – supervised
   f = individual – unsupervised

E. Type of activity:
   a = play
   b = directed
   c = directed/choice of two
   d = free choice

F. Relationships and social interaction:
   a = initiates conversation with adult
   b = initiates conversation with peer
   c = interacts positively with adult concerning task/activity
   d = interacts positively with peer concerning task/activity
   e = shows concern towards adult
   f = shows concern towards peer
   g = responds positively towards approach from adult
   h = responds positively towards approach from peer
   i = rejects approach from adult
   j = rejects approach from peer
   k = deliberately distracts peer
   l = deliberately disrupts peer's work
   m = shows aggression towards adult
   n = shows aggression towards peer
   o = no interaction

Times (m/s)	D	E	F
0/0			
0/10			
0/20			
0/30			
0/40			
0/50			
1/0			
1/10			
1/20			
1/30			
1/40			
1/50			
2/0			
2/10			
2/20			
2/30			
2/40			
2/50			
3/0			
3/10			
3/20			
3/30			
3/40			
3/50			
4/0			

APPENDIX 6
Additional Reference Resources and Materials

Videos

1. *Good Companions* (Sherborne, 1986)
   Veronica Sherborne's last video shows her way of working with pupils and students across a spectrum of special educational needs.
   Available from: Concord Video and Film Council Ltd, Rosehill Centre, 22 Hines Road, Ipswich, Suffolk, UK, IP3 9BG. Tel. +44 (0)1473 726012

2. *Never Say Never* (Hill, 1998)
   Cyndi Hill's video, illustrating the use of Sherborne Developmental Movement with varying groups of pupils and students, focuses on the implementation of Sherborne's ideas in the context of its underpinning philosophical perspectives.
   Available from: twotors@hotmail.com

3. *With Too Much Falling and Getting Up*
   This video shows stages of natural development in the child from 0–3 years. The absence of these stages is an indication of possible problems.
   Available, with English 'voice over', from:
   SIG Educational Centre, Kerkham 1-2, B-9070 Destelbergen, Belgium
   Tel. +32 (0)9 238 3125; Fax +32 (0)9 238 3140; email: info@sig-net.be

4. *A View of Developmental Movement, Based on the Work of Veronica Sherborne* (Bontinck and Van Daele, 2004)
   This is an introduction to Veronica Sherborne and her early work. It shows examples of SDM with groups of varying ages and abilities. This is a 'taster' video to encourage interested people to pursue the training courses offered by the Sherborne Associations.
   Available, with English 'voice over', from:
   SIG Educational Centre, Kerkham 1-2, B-9070 Destelbergen, Belgium
   Tel. +32 (0)9 238 3125; Fax +32 (0)9 238 3140; email: info@sig-net.be

A list of Sherborne Developmental Movement materials, course information and access details can be found on
The Sherborne Association UK website
www.sherborne-association.org.uk

Index

Accelerated Learning,	22, 23, 24
affective climate,	52
aggression,	13, 41, 53, 67, 84, 127
altruism,	16, 17, 27 – 29, 91, 102, 113
analysis:	
of data,	114, 121
of movement,	see 'Laban'
assessment,	35, 41, 46, 57, 142 – 152
attachment,	22, 52, 53
attention,	16, 26, 32, 72 – 79, 84, 85, 87 – 89, 112, 114, 119, 153
Attention Deficit/Hyperactivity Disorder (ADHD),	41, 46, 49
autistic spectrum disorder (ASD),	12, 28, 42, 46 – 47, 49, 62, 102, 103, 105, 108, 110, 119 – 121
autonomy,	74, 91
awareness of self and others,	3, 7, 10, 15, 17, 20, 21, 27 – 29, 32, 36, 38, 40, 41, 45, 55, 63 – 66, 75, 76, 82 – 90, 97, 101, 104, 113, 120, 124, 126–152
beneficial aspects,	xiv, 9, 13 – 17, 20, 28, 32, 40, 43, 45, 48, 58 – 60, 63 – 66, 74, 92, 95 – 98, 102, 103, 113 – 119, 123
blanket play,	35, 42 – 47, 103, 139
body awareness,	see 'awareness of self and others'
bonding,	51 – 61
broadening perspective,	xv, 51*ff*, 123–124
Bruner:	
scaffolding,	30 – 31, 59
centring,	64, 66 – 67, 72, 85, 128, 129, 133 – 134
children in charge,	31, 90
cognitive development,	26, 28, 52, 74, 118 – 119
communication:	15 – 17, 21, 23, 31, 35 – 37, 47, 51 – 53, 59, 69 – 70, 72, 76 – 80, 82, 84, 113, 120, 123
body language,	11, 36 – 37, 71, 77, 84
facial expression,	77, 84
gesture,	39, 76, 77, 78, 84
movement language,	52, 97 – 98
non-verbal communication,	17, 36 – 37, 54, 76 – 77, 79, 84
verbal/communication,	36, 38, 53, 72, 74, 75, 76 – 79, 84 – 85
vocalisation,	36
competency,	15, 22, 30, 31, 52, 71, 74, 97
concentration,	16, 26 – 27, 41, 66, 72, 74, 84, 89, 101, 114 – 119, 127, 153
confidence,	3, 5 10, 11, 13, 14 – 16, 24 – 26, 27, 32, 48, 52, 53, 55, 57, 71 – 75, 84, 86, 88, 89 – 91, 94 – 98, 102, 104, 126, 127
contents of a session,	38 – 42
courses,	70, 79, 82, 155
creativity,	12, 14, 16, 23, 24, 36, 37, 38, 59, 67, 88, 89, 102, 104, 126, 151 – 152

dance,	2 – 3, 51 – 68, 89, 91, 101, 108 – 111
danger,	63
developmental aspects,	5, 7, 8, 9, 10, 15, 16, 17 – 18, 19 – 22, 26 – 27, 28 – 32, 43 – 45,
	57, 59, 69 – 79, 88, 91, 102, 112, 113, 118 – 119, 127, 155
Developmental Play,	17, 51 – 61
differentiation,	14
early intervention,	22, 51 – 61, 120
early years,	44, 51 – 61
educators,	70
emotion,	11, 12 – 13, 16, 22, 25 – 26, 31, 36, 44, 49, 52, 55, 59, 72, 77, 84, 92 – 97
emotional development,	22, 44, 74, 91
energy,	13, 26, 38, 40, 49, 54, 55, 63, 64, 66 – 67, 72, 73, 84, 86 – 87, 105
enjoyment,	14, 16, 25, 43, 50, 52, 54, 62, 66, 67, 70 – 71, 80, 101 – 102, 110
equality,	2, 11, 12, 14, 28, 70, 71 – 74, 78, 92, 93, 106, 127
evolving theory,	7*ff*, 125
excitement,	22, 63
expertise,	70
eye-contact,	46, 47, 53, 63, 66, 71, 77, 84, 103
Feuerstein:	
Instrumental Enrichment,	21, 22, 25, 26
Flanders Interaction Analysis Categories (FIAC),	114
flexibility,	12, 14, 38, 40, 47, 102, 104
floor,	11, 12, 36, 38, 41, 42, 43, 45, 47, 49, 55, 103, 103 – 106, 128 – 141
fun,	10, 14, 16, 25, 52, 54, 63, 65, 70 – 71, 78, 80, 96–97, 105
functional independence,	74
goals,	12, 22, 32, 69, 70, 71, 76 – 77, 79, 93, 97
Higher Education (HE),	48, 93 – 99
holistic approach,	52, 69
hyperactivity,	41, 46, 49, 105
implementation,	xiii, xv, 8, 10 – 11, 13 – 15, 18, 31, 46 – 50, 91, 92, 102 – 103, 110, 112, 123 – 124, 125, 155
inclusion,	x, xiv, 17, 92 – 93, 96, 98
insecurity,	12, 27, 44
interaction,	8, 10, 11, 13, 15, 16, 17, 20 – 22, 25, 27, 29, 30, 38, 44, 52, 54, 57, 62 – 68, 77 – 79, 112 – 118, 120, 154
international,	5, 69 – 79, 118, 123
interpersonal skills,	15, 16, 19, 31, 55, 91, 92, 102
issues,	xiii, xv, 42 – 45, 49, 91, 102 – 103

key words,	13 – 14, 22 – 24, 73
Laban:	2 – 9, 39, 72, 77, 84, 95, 108
'free dance',	2, 110
movement analysis,	2 – 4, 39, 108
movement qualities,	3 – 5, 38, 39, 72, 75, 104, 126
language,	15 – 16, 36, 38, 48, 51, 71, 72, 75, 76 – 79, 85, 97 – 98
learning environment,	42, 57, 93, 102
levels of support,	31, 32, 49
mental health,	59 – 60
MISC programme,	22
mixed ability,	10, 14, 35, 37, 42, 106, 55, 93, 155
moderate learning difficulties,	62, 64
motor:	
cognition,	70, 72
control,	70
development,	70 – 74, 98
movement expeiences,	2, 5, 7, 8, 9, 10, 14, 15, 16, 17, 21, 27, 32, 36, 37, 40, 41, 42, 46, 47, 48, 49, 52, 53, 63 – 64, 65–67, 71, 75, 85, 89, 97 – 98, 101, 104, 105, 106, 108, 128 – 141
movement play,	17, 51 – 59
multidisciplinary team,	69, 70, 73
muscle tone,	72
music,	42, 64, 89, 91, 101, 108 – 110
National Curriculum:	82 – 99
access to,	17, 47
English,	84
Mathematics,	85
PE,	88 – 89, 96 – 97
PSHE and Citizenship	90
Science,	86 – 87
non-prescriptive,	12, 14, 16, 24
nurses,	70
objective analysis,	xii
observation,	2, 3, 7, 14, 35, 37, 41, 54, 57, 58, 59, 71, 74, 77, 78, 86, 112 – 118, 121, 142 – 152, 153 – 154
occupational therapy,	73 – 75
parents,	2, 22, 45, 51 – 61, 69 – 71, 80, 103, 114, 118
pedagogy,	x, 11
peer-group partners,	13, 31, 65 – 67
person-centred approach,	14
personal development,	27, 29, 35, 45, 83, 102, 107, 124
philosophical considerations,	20 – 22
physical contact,	35, 41 – 42, 44 – 45, 52, 71, 103, 106, 124

physical disabilities,	16, 42, 43, 47 – 48, 49, 91, 106
physiotherapy,	42, 70 – 73, 80 – 81, 103
Piaget,	29 – 30, 74 – 75
play,	16, 17, 28, 31, 40, 42, 50, 51, 69 – 70, 71, 72, 74, 75, 78 – 79, 80, 94, 113, 127
positive experience,	11, 14, 23, 25, 32, 37, 53, 58, 60, 75, 91, 102
post-natal depression,	59
practical aspects,	xii, 35 – 50, 54, 102 – 103, 106, 123
practice,	6, 8, 9, 10, 18, 34*ff*, 51, 52, 54, 55, 92, 96
praise,	12, 27, 37, 66, 90
profound and multiple learning difficulties (PMLD),	36, 43, 46, 47, 49, 80, 82 – 83, 92, 93, 103
progression,	10, 15, 17, 31, 35, 36, 39, 46, 50, 65, 67, 70, 77, 88, 90, 98, 128 – 141
psychological implications,	xiv, 4, 7, 9, 17, 19 – 20, 22 – 24, 27 – 29, 74, 79, 124
psychologists,	20, 23, 70, 95, 123
psychomotor therapy,	72 – 73
QCA Guidelines,	83 – 93
quality:	
of interaction,	xv, 11, 21, 25, 30, 60, 78, 118
of learning experience,	xvi, 11
of movement,	3 – 4, 38, 39, 63, 65, 71, 97, 151 – 152
questions/answers,	8, 11, 13, 15, 101 – 107, 125
recording:	
video,	35 – 36, 59, 60, 106, 121, 155
written,	35 – 36, 59, 113, 115 – 116, 121, 142 – 152
relationships,	3, 5, 7, 14, 15, 16, 17, 24, 25, 28, 31, 38, 39, 43, 44, 51 – 61, 62, 64, 66, 67, 71, 75, 76, 77, 79, 90, 91, 94, 95, 102, 111, 114, 118, 119, 120, 126, 127, 147 – 150
relationship work:	12, 13, 24, 28, 29, 36, 38, 41, 43, 49, 72, 86, 90, 92, 104, 113, 127
'against',	9, 13, 26, 41, 58, 63 – 65, 66, 73, 84, 86, 90, 126, 127, 129, 136, 139, 140
'shared',	9, 58, 63 – 64, 71, 73, 126, 127, 130, 136, 140
'with/caring',	9, 58, 62, 66, 72 – 73, 75, 84, 86, 90, 127, 129, 132 – 133, 135, 138, 139
relaxation,	36, 38, 42, 53, 63, 64, 94, 96, 130, 136
research,	17, 23, 26 – 27, 29, 31, 47, 59, 112 – 122, 124, 125
respect,	11, 12, 15, 17, 20, 24, 29, 40, 43, 54, 55, 65, 66, 70, 71, 98, 106
responsibility,	21, 43, 45, 55, 63, 66, 69, 84, 90, 91, 93, 127
risk,	15, 43
role:	
of child/participant,	12, 14, 28 – 29, 31, 32, 71, 76, 84, 90, 91, 93, 127
of care-giver/helper/supporter,	9, 11 – 13, 15, 20, 21, 24, 25, 27, 28 – 31, 35, 37, 38, 42 – 43, 46, 63–64, 70, 78, 95, 103, 106
of teacher,	see 'teacher approach' and 'knowledge'
rolling,	9, 18, 39, 49, 50, 58, 62 – 63, 67, 69, 72, 85, 86, 88, 89, 105, 108, 109, 128 – 139

Index

safety of:
- *environment,* 42 – 43, 52, 57, 92
- *equipment,* 45, 103, 106
- *helpers/supporters,* 42, 43, 46 – 47, 48, 52 – 53, 63, 103
- *participants,* 42 – 43, 45, 46 – 47, 52 – 53, 63

security, 12, 13, 16, 17, 24 – 26, 31, 44, 46, 50, 52, 53, 54, 55, 58, 72, 73, 74, 82, 84, 95

self:
- *awareness,* 7, 8, 20, 21, 27, 29, 37, 55, 64, 66, 72, 75, 86, 87, 90, 94, 126
- *concept,* 16, 17, 20, 27, 55, 58, 63, 66, 79, 90, 124
- *confidence,* 10, 11, 14 – 15, 16, 27, 52, 55, 58, 71, 74, 94, 95, 98, 102, 126, 127
- *esteem,* 10, 11, 14, 16, 17, 24, 27, 37, 52, 58, 66, 67, 74, 75, 88, 90, 102
- *expression,* 5, 8, 37, 91
- *image,* 10, 14, 16, 17, 19, 23, 25, 27, 60, 86, 94, 102, 126
- *respect,* 55
- *worth,* 10, 21, 27, 55, 58

sensitivity, 5, 11, 13, 15, 16, 27, 28, 29, 32, 44, 46, 50, 52, 53, 54, 58, 64, 71, 72, 78, 88, 90, 95, 97, 102, 111, 113, 120, 127

severe learning difficulties 7, 14, 19, 40, 49, 82 – 83, 89, 92, 108, 114, 120

shared experience, 2, 7, 8, 9, 10, 11, 12, 14, 21, 25, 28, 29, 31, 32, 37, 39, 40, 41, 42, 47, 52, 60, 64, 66, 71, 77, 84, 88, 89, 90, 98, 113, 124

Sherborne, Veronica:
- *Biography and context,* 2 – 5
- *tributes,* 5

Sherborne Developmental Movement (SDM):
- *definition,* 8
- *title,* 7 – 8

SDM activities: 128 – 141
- *'rocks'* 64
- *starting/finishing a session,* 41 – 42, 46, 103, 104, 105, 110

SDM in:
- *dance,* 51 – 61, 62 – 68
- *edcuation,* 82 – 99, 108 – 111, 112 – 119
- *family therapy,* 51 – 61
- *projects,* 108 – 111
- *research,* 112 – 122

social:
- *context,* 25, 29, 31, 79, 95, 98
- *development,* 15, 16, 17, 18, 22, 24, 28 – 33, 44, 63, 74, 75, 77 – 78, 79, 113 – 114, 118 – 119
- *effectiveness,* 72
- *engagement,* 47, 119 – 121
- *interaction,* 16 – 17, 27, 29, 63, 64, 77, 113 – 114, 117, 120, 154
- *skills,* 51, 64, 66 – 67, 92

159

space,	5, 10, 12, 38 – 39, 47, 72, 73, 84, 85, 88, 89, 97, 104, 108 – 109, 128 – 139
spatial awareness,	3 – 4, 16, 17, 38, 75, 80, 85 – 88, 126, 145 – 146
speech and language therapy,	70, 73, 76 – 79
stress,	23, 60
success,	8, 13, 16, 21, 22 – 24, 25, 27, 30, 32, 37, 46, 54, 58, 73, 74, 90, 95, 102, 124
tactile defensiveness,	42, 46, 47, 49, 71, 103, 106
'TAMBA',	63 – 64
teachers,	21, 24, 27, 50, 53, 54, 83
teacher approach and qualities,	3, 11 – 13, 12, 20 – 25, 27, 37, 42, 43, 50, 52, 54, 57, 101, 103, 104, 106, 138 – 139
teaching style,	11, 12, 21, 24, 25, 92, 106
team building,	23, 48, 94
themes,	12, 38, 89, 108–111
timing,	40 – 42
touch,	13, 35, 43 – 45, 52–53, 64 – 65, 71, 95, 101, 103, 155
toys,	75, 76, 78 – 79
trust,	5, 10, 11, 12 – 13, 14, 15, 16, 26, 48, 52, 53, 55, 69, 71, 74, 75, 94, 98, 102, 113, 126, 127, 132, 135, 139
turn-taking,	22, 40, 49, 63, 77, 78, 79, 127
uniqueness,	52
valuing people,	11 – 12, 14, 24, 44, 90, 92 – 93, 98, 106
varying needs,	42, 46 – 49, 70
vulnerability,	44, 64, 95
Vygotsky:	
zone of proximal development,	30
warm up,	62, 65
wheelchairs,	43, 62